ESSENTIAL OILS

The Guide to Get Started With Essential Oils

(The Young Living Book Guide of Natural Remedies for Beginners for Pets)

Karmen Price

Published By Darby Connor

Karmen Price

All Rights Reserved

Essential Oils: The Guide to Get Started With Essential Oils (The Young Living Book Guide of Natural Remedies for Beginners for Pets)

ISBN 978-1-77485-322-1

All rights reserved. No part of this guide may be reproduced in any form without permission in writing from the publisher except in the case of brief quotations embodied in critical articles or reviews.

Legal & Disclaimer

The information contained in this book is not designed to replace or take the place of any form of medicine or professional medical advice. The information in this book has been provided for educational and entertainment purposes only.

The information contained in this book has been compiled from sources deemed reliable, and it is accurate to the best of the Author's knowledge; however, the Author cannot guarantee its accuracy and validity and cannot be held liable for any errors or omissions. Changes are periodically made to this book. You must consult your doctor or get professional medical advice before using any of the suggested remedies, techniques, or information in this book.

Upon using the information contained in this book, you agree to hold harmless the Author from and against any damages, costs, and expenses, including any legal fees potentially resulting from the application of any of the information provided by this guide. This disclaimer applies to any damages or injury caused by the use and application, whether directly or indirectly, of any advice or information presented, whether for breach of contract, tort, negligence, personal injury, criminal intent, or under any other cause of action.

You agree to accept all risks of using the information presented inside this book. You need to consult a professional medical practitioner in order to ensure you are both able and healthy enough to participate in this program.

TABLE OF CONTENTS

INTRODUCTION 1

CHAPTER 1: UNDERSTANDING ESSENTIAL OILS 4

CHAPTER 2: SHORT BACKGROUND OF ESSENTIAL OILS.... 10

CHAPTER 3: STRESS REDUCTION 16

CHAPTER 4: LEARNING TO BE AWARE OF ESSENTIAL OILS 27

CHAPTER 5: WEIGHT LOSS ESSENTIAL OILS RECIPES 35

CHAPTER 6: OILS ESSENTIAL FOR ARTHRITIS PAIN 38

CHAPTER 7: OIL PULLING WITH ESSENTIAL OILS 47

CHAPTER 8: THE ESSENTIAL OIL AND STRESS 51

CHAPTER 9: THE ESSENTIAL OILS THAT ARE SAFE FOR CHILDREN 56

CHAPTER 10: INCREASING MARKET THE RISE OF ESSENTIAL OILS 74

CHAPTER 11: ESSENTIAL OILS: ALL ABOUT 83

CHAPTER 12: ESSENTIAL OILS FOR SLEEP DISORDERS & TRANQUILITY 94

CHAPTER 13: BENEFITS OF ESSENTIAL OILS 102

CHAPTER 14: WHAT TO TAKE CARE OF YOUR ESSENTIAL OILS 109

CHAPTER 15: THE POWER OF SMELL 114

CHAPTER 16: PURCHASE AND STORING ESSENTIAL OILS 124

CHAPTER 17: EUCALYPTUS OIL 137

CHAPTER 18: THE ESSENTIAL OILS AND THEIR BENEFICIAL EFFECTS 144

CHAPTER 19: NUTMEG ESSENTIAL OIL 170

CONCLUSION 180

Introduction

That's the reason this book came to be - I've put together a collection of dishes that are ready for use . All the recipes included in the cookbook have passed a rigorous test for effectiveness as well as safety and are ready to use.

There are recipes to clean your home, to help to treat minor illnesses and to boost your immunity, keep the skin glowing, for babies and mommy, for the big brother and little sister and even for your pet in the family - this is a cookbook packed with recipes to help keep your loved ones healthier, more attractive and more content overall.

All you have to do is select the category you are interested in and select the recipe you like most. Then, gather the ingredients and prepare the recipe in your own kitchen.

If you're just beginning in the field of essential oils in your home, this guide provides recipes created by professional aromatherapists over time and step-by-step directions to follow. Imagine it as an extensive cheat sheet you can reap all the benefits, without having to be concerned about making mistakes or wasting time.

If however you know a bit about the way essential oils function and the properties they possess You don't have to read everything over again. This book is ideal for you. It's filled with recipes you can attempt at your own pace, without the explanations you've seen hundreds of times before.

If you're a novice or an experienced cook This book will offer fresh recipes you can explore and enjoy

The goal is to give you recipes you can make and therefore, we've left out sections on safety procedures. So I recommend that you follow the recipes exactly as they are described in the book. You should make any substitutions only if you know the basics of mixing essential oil blends and how to stay safe when making use of essential oils.

Essential oils are powerful and when used in the right dilutions, can prove to be a very useful instrument. If they are used in dilutions which are excessive, however it is possible for problems to arise.

If you are feeling that you'd like to alter the recipes, I recommend to make sure that the dilutions are the same that you make it a triple or double recipe, if you want but maintain the basic recipe.

If you're looking to exchange one oil to another, I suggest to conduct additional research on how to blend oils, particularly in the case of oils that are used on children or pet.

Chapter 1: Understanding Essential Oils

Over the years, the essential oils were utilized for various reasons. They are used for their cosmetic benefits and also for their spiritual and emotional benefits. Essential oils are extracted liquid that comes from different components of a plant, and generally have the properties of the plant it was made from and more. If they are extracted using a meticulous steam distillation technique or what's called cold pressing which is the purest form of essential oils are thought to be more potent than the plants that they originally extracted.

The advantages of essential oils vary from weight loss and cleansing to supporting all systems of the body. They offer the answers needed to restore balance and to feel at their most optimal. Essential oils are generally very concentrated and only some are always highly beneficial. The main distinction with perfumes and essential oils is essential oils must be extracted from plants, while perfume oils don't contain natural ingredients and aren't able to provide beneficial benefits for health. Essential oils are able to be beneficial throughout your daily life.

The essential oil you choose is contingent on the intended use and you must conduct a thorough study by speaking with experienced people. You can also purchase an aromatherapy book that focuses on therapeutic. Always be aware of the warnings that come with the specific oil and way to apply it. It is important to know that essential oils are absorbed into the body through three ways i.e. applied via the skin or swallowed and the method used to apply them is based on the effect you want to achieve and the kind of essential oil chosen. Essential oils are in various ways for centuries e.g. the reduction of stress, they aid in increasing your concentration, they assist to relax your muscles, cleanse the body, aid to maintain the emotional equilibrium of the body and help to boost your body's immune system. The majority of essential oils have antiseptic properties , but some are also distinguished by anti-fungal, antiviral, and antibacterial properties.

The benefits and uses of essential oils

Essential oils were utilized over the years for their medicinal health, as well as other reasons. The uses of essential oils range from cleaning products to natural medicinal treatments, personal beauty products and aromatherapy. However, if anyone uses essential oils, they should be aware of security precautions and use the oils in a safe manner.

The advantages of essential oils stem from their antioxidant, antimicrobial an antibacterial, antiviral, anti-fungal as well as anti-inflammatory qualities. Essential oils are becoming increasingly well-known because they are natural treatments that don't come with any negative side negative effects. There are many benefits associated with essential oils . I will only mention just a few which are

1.)They are simple, convenient and simple to utilize. They are able to be used wherever e.g. at work, home in the daytime, and they can be carried everywhere.

2.)Essential oils aid in aromatherapy massage. They aid us in dealing minor aches and pains which may result from day to everyday activities.

3.)Because they're taken from plants, they do not have any harmful effects as long as you only use one kind of essential oil to its intended use e.g. essential oils used for home use are not suitable for human use.

4.)They easily penetrate cell membranes and the skin. Essential oils are able to easily pass through the brain barrier to

access lympic areas of the brain that regulate beliefs, moods and emotions. This can help you beat anger, stress, and other emotional issues.

5.)Essential oils can help soothe the skin and soothe irritation, rejuvenate it and strengthen your immune system.

6.)Essential oils possess oxygen-enhancing properties that permit them to transfer essential nutrients directly to the cells nutrient-deficient or oxygen deficient.

7.)Essential oils are antioxidants that boosts the health of the body and assists in preventing harm from environmental factors, aging, and diet.

8.)Essential oils improve digestion and aids in easing digestion.

9.)Essential oils are also used in making homemade lotions, such as shampoos and shower gels, perfumes soaps, facial toners and many other natural products.

10.)They are also employed for freshening up rooms and general freshening of the home.

Physical characteristics of essential oils

1.)They are very scent-filled, concentrated, and powerful ingredients.

2.)They are not oily in texture since they are not fat-based.

3.)They are able to evaporate easily into air and therefore are highly volatile.

4.)Essential oils are prone to heat, and must be kept in a cool, dry area.

5.)They can also be sensitive to sunlight, and should be kept in dark bottles.

6.)They aren't able to dissolve in water.

7.)All essential oils contain antibacterial properties.

Chapter 2: Short Background of Essential Oils

Essential oils are described as a natural oil that is typically produced by distillation that is carried out by a plant another source to make an oil that has the distinctive aroma of the plant. Oils that are essential have been utilized to serve a myriad of reasons all over the globe for many thousands of years. The earliest indications of the medicinal properties of plants were discovered in France and go back as far back as one-hundred years ago BCE (20,000 decades ago)! Even our ancestors knew the healing properties of plants that can be used for a myriad of issues.

In the case of plant oils The earliest evidence of their usage dates back to Egypt around 4500 BCE. The use of these oils was element of the daily life of Egypt and they utilized the oils and extracts from plants for cosmetics, medicine and to treat medical issues. Essential oils were also used during their ceremonies of worship and each scent was sacred to the gods. They would then apply anointing to the statues of these goddesses and gods in their worship services and give them respect. It did not seem that the Egyptians created themselves essential oils. Instead they imported oils from other areas.

China as well as India are two nations where people have used essential oils for a long time. China also has written evidence of the use of essential oils. The Yellow Emperor, Huang Ti wrote a book entitled the Yellow Emperor's Book of Internal Medicine, that detailed their use. A lot of the practices used by oils from China many thousands of years ago are being practiced to this day. They have been tested for time. In India the oil was used to make healing potion and evidence of these actions indicating that they began around 3000 years ago.

The father of Modern Medicine, Hypocrites of the Greek civilization recorded the therapeutic effects of around 300 plants used for essential oil. The majority of his information on these plants from Egyptians as well as the Indians prior to his time. A lot of the information comes be obtained from exchange of information during the time that Greek soldiers came across people on the Indian subcontinent on their way to travel along with Alexander the Great.

The hypocrites advised that people take "a fragranced bath and aromatic massage each day is the best way to achieve healthy living." (From His writings). His writings later were influential to the Romans and led to Marcus Aurelius, a Roman emperor, locating a amount of information on health, such as essential oils, in his writings.

In the past, the use of essential oils was widely practiced in Rome for all. The use of oils and fragrances was common in massages and baths by the common people, and were believed to boost overall wellness and health.

At the present it was the herbs and flowers in themselves that were utilized in the production of the scents and potions as well as the medications that were utilized. It was actually the Persian named Ali-Ibn Saa, who was also popularly known as Avicenna the Arab who first came across and wrote down the procedure to distill essential oils in the way they are in the present. He was a doctor who wrote a work on the health benefits of approximately 800 plants, as well as their effects on human health. The information he shared is still used to this day.

In the Crusades during the Crusades, people from Europe gained a lot of knowledge about Persian methods of distilling essential oils. They then brought their knowledge and methods back to the home country and spread across all over the European continent. The 14th century was when it was reported that people utilized Frankincense and Pine to fight off the "evil spirits" which they believed caused their Bubonic Plague. It is not surprising that documents show that there were less deaths from the disease in areas that were a part of this practice.

Authors from Europe such as Nicholas Culpeper (16753) and Ren-Maurice Gattesfosse, a chemist (1928) published articles on the therapeutic properties of plants as well as its essential oils. The book written by Culpeper, The Complete Herbal and Gattesfosse's book Aromatherapie both have had an impact on the medical practices in Europe and were later translated to American.

As you can observe from this short history that the healing and therapeutic properties of herbs have been recognized since the beginning of time, and revisited by each generation, and knowledge is distributed throughout the globe. If essential oils didn't work, the understanding of them would have vanished into obscurity. However, the opposite occurred. Due to the healing properties that these herbs possess, new methods of using them become known, like distilling essential oils. These essential oils can be employed for a variety of purposes. This chapter is going to discuss about the application of essential oils to help you lose weight. In the next chapter, we'll talk about the most important things you should be aware of to make use of this amazing tool to achieve your weight loss goals.

Chapter 3: Stress Reduction

Methods of Diffusion

A lot of the things that are used to diffuse are items that you already have at your home. Make use of a diffuser to bring an aroma that is natural to your house and set the right mood. It can aid in concentration as well as insomnia. It can also with some illnesses.

There's a product that you can utilize in any area in your home that requires an extra dose of freshness. It's safe for all, including children. It is only a tiny amount of oil could be absorbed by your body during the process of diffusion.

Candle Diffusion

Find a beeswax or a soy candle and allow it to burn for five minutes or as long. Blowing the candle out, add a drop of oil to the wax that has been melted (not the burning wick). Light the candle again and take pleasure in. Take extra care as the mixture is extremely inflammable.

You can also buy an oil diffuser for candles that utilizes an electric tealight to warm the oil. The diffuser is designed with an opening in which an empty bowl or tray can be able to fit. There are many various shapes and colors to match your interior. In most cases there is no need for electricity. Always carry a spare cord in case your device has an electrical cord.

Tissue Diffusion

The scent is easily transferred to any area inside your home. Add 2 to 3 drops of your oil of choice on a paper. You can also use it when you're in an airplane or in a workplace cubicle. But, you won't take in the aromas of the entire area, only in the area that the tissue is situated.

Lamp Ring Diffusers

The majority of lamp ring designs are constructed out of brass or terracotta designed to look like a ring. It is glued directly to the bulb. The scent is dispersed throughout the space. Make sure you follow the directions of the manufacturer. The oils could damage the bulb if properly handled.

Steam Diffusion

Pour 2 cups of water that is boiling in an container. Add up to 10 drops of the oil. You can enjoy this any time at any time, whether all day or night. The steam will soon be released into the room, but not stay for long.

Electric Heat Diffusers

Larger areas can be covered by the use of an electrical unit dependent on the design and model. Electrical units are also able to effectively disperse thicker oils like Patchouli or Sandalwood. Alcohol will usually aid in the dissolution of any residue left inside the unit.

Ultrasonic Diffusers

Water and ultrasonic wave diffusion essential oils you prefer in your office or home space. You can select from a range of sizes and styles. Some of them may even have lighting that is colored to enhance. The availability of these units is increasing widespread because they're so cost-effective. Some models can also supply humidity to the room if required. It is essential to follow the directions of the user carefully to get the most effective outcomes.

Cool Air Nebulizing Diffusers

The therapeutic benefits are optimized to ensure an optimal impact. It is also possible to wear the terracotta pendant necklace diffuser. If you're looking to scent an aroma you love, it's right there.

Two Diffusers, specially for the Christmas Season

Happy Holidays!

What to Do:

1 drop Wintergreen

2 drops of each of white and wild orange the fir

Choose one of these combinations on your fabric or any other technique you prefer.

The Candy Store

What to Utilize:

2 drops of each of wintergreen and wild orange essential oils

Simply add the oils you want in an opaque glass bottle and make a unique blend for you. The process of experimentation is an excellent method to find your preferred fragrances, so you should start with small amounts first , before you increase on the amount.

Diffuser Blends:

Use the recommended drops to create your unique scent:

Blend 1:2 Bergamot 4 , each of Ylang Ylang & Clary Sage

Blend 2 Blend 2 Vanilla | 1 Ylang Ylang

Blend 3 Blend 3: Blend 3: Sweet Orange |1 Jasmine3 Patchouli

Blend 4: 10 Lime |2 Ylang Ylang |1 Rose | 7 Bergamot

Blend 5 Blend 5: 9 Sandalwood1 Neroli

Blend 6 Blend 6: 2. Scotch Pine|1 Rose 2 lemon Sandalwood

Blend 7:9 5 each from Lavender & Spearmint

Blend 3 Sweet Oranges Jasmine and Cinnamon

Blend 9:11 Lemon Bergamot 3 Spearmint

Blend 10:12 Patchouli 5 drops Vanilla1 Neroli 2 Linden Blossom

Blend 11: 1 Roman Chamomile|5 Rosemary|3 Lavender|1 Peppermint

Blend 12 Blend 12: 4 Bergamot 3 Sandalwood1 Jasmine2 Grapefruit

Blend 13 Blend 13: 5 Bergamot 1 Cypress 4 Lavender

Blend 14: 5 Lavender|1 Ylang Ylang |4 Rosewood

Blend 15 Blend 15 Grapefruit Two each from Lemon as well as Ylang Ylang

Mix 16: 1 Cinnamon 3 Sweet Orange Juniper

Healthy Spray to use before bed for Monsters

Although it isn't an oil you apply to your body, it does earn as a scents for bedtime. Some people have referred to it as "Shoo the Monsters Away spray.

Try this mix:

30 d. emulsifier

8 d. Orange

12 . d. of each of the following:

Lavender

Roman Chamomile

8-ounce bottle of base room spray

Mixing the Ingredients:

Mix the oils together with the base and emulsifier. Shake thoroughly.

How to Utilize:

Simply spray them away and let the room smell fresh. Spray a little on your pillow for additional enjoyment.

Bay Oil

A strong scent similar to clove oil is evident in this oil. It can be used as a massage oil , or use it in burners or vaporizers. Small amounts of it can create an euphoric effect, while more oil could cause the effect of sedation.

It can be useful for the following:

Depression

What to Do:

1 tbsp. of Jojoba Oil

2 2. from Bay Oil

4. each of the following:

Black Pepper

Bergamot Oil

Relaxation:

What to Utilize:

10 d. Bay Oil

1 d. Clove EO

2 to 3 2 to 3. 2 to 3 d.

Almond Oil for the carrier oil

Stress Reduction

A study conducted in 2013 found that the smell of lavender, chamomile and neroli can be beneficial in reducing anxiety and stress.

Use this method:

3 . each of the following:

Lavender

Marjoram

To 15 ml, add 15 ml unscented Lotion

Mix the ingredients to relax the muscles that are tight and relax your stressed mind.

Enjoy a relaxing massage

The Aphrodisiac Blend

What to Utilize:

2. Jasmine

8 d. Sandalwood

To Treat Sore Muscles

What to Do:

5. Eucalyptus

4 d. Peppermint

1 d. Black Pepper

2 d. Ginger

The Stress Buster

What to Utilize:

3 d. Lavender

2 d. Lemon

6 D. Clary Sage

How to prepare Mix the oils you want to use and store them in an airtight, dark glass container.

To Apply: Use just 1/2-1/2 teaspoon for massage.

Chapter 4: Learning to Be Aware of Essential oils

The first step to unleash the potential that essential oils have is to understand the nature of them and how they work and how you can use the right way.

Which essential oils are they?

Essential oils are the essential oils found in plants. To clarify, "essential" refers to the extracts of essences from plants or specific plant components. Chemically the plant is made up of 3 elements including water, plant fiber , or cellulose, and its essential nutrients, or its essence. The essence is extracted from the plant by boiling it, and distilling the tea, or by squeezeing the plant before further distilling the juice. The essence of the plant is what makes it a specific plant. Without it any plant will have the same chemical form.

The second, "oil" refers to the fact that essential oils are hydrophobic, that means they don't combine with water. Shaking vigorously will cause the essential oil to mix and water. However, in the end they will split.

What are essential oils able to be used for or are they employed to do? Essential oils can perform whatever the plant does. For instance, smelling the lavender plant may relax the nerves. Thus, snuffing an essential lavender oil can have the similar effects. In the end, it's the essential ingredient of lavender that provides the relaxing effect. The one difference between the lavender plant and its essential oil is that the latter's concentration.

How can essential oils be utilized?

It is important to note that essential oils aren't only artificially fragranced oils, which some untrustworthy manufacturers prefer to refer to as "essential oils." These synthetic fragrance oils, like the names suggest, synthetic while essential oils are entirely natural. If you're using essential oils to provide nutrients for plants and not for the scent that they provide, then synthetic fragrance oils is ineffective. In contrast when you use essential oils solely for their scent, then you could manage using premium synthetic fragrance oils. However, people with more sophisticated senses may claim that the scent of their oils is less appealing. This topic will be covered more in the subsequent chapters.

To determine if you're buying genuine essential oil or synthetic fragrance oil, you must check the cost. The former is more expensive in comparison to the latter due to the way it is made. It is important to remember that a plant is composed of cellulose, water and the essence of it. The majority of the plant's content is composed of cellulose and water. This means that you will need many plants to extract a tiny volume of essential oils. For instance, it requires around eleven pounds of lavender in order to produce just 15 milliliters of essential oil. In light of the time and effort involved in growing the lavender plant as well as the labor involved in extraction of the oil will not be logical to pay just $1 for 15 milliliters of essential lavender oil (unless it is, of course, the shop is having an enormous sale.)

An acceptable price for most common essential oils, like lavender is around 10 dollars per 30 milliliter. The more uncommon essential oils like frankincense are likely to cost more because there aren't any manufacturers manufacture these. The cost will also be contingent on the difficulty to obtain the oil, and/or the difficulty to cultivate the plant. Additionally the essential oil taken by organically-grown plants can twice the cost due to the difficulties that organic farming brings.

To make sure you're receiving genuine essential oils ensure that you are buying from trusted brands and retailers. The oils are sold in bottles properly labeled that contain that the name scientifically used for the plant and the country from which it originated or the place where the plant was grown as well as the year of its manufacture. They also sell essential oils in opaque, dark bottles that block light from destroying the oil. The label should indicate what the essence oil was dilute or not. The reasons behind why purchasing dilute essential oils could be beneficial will be covered in the subsequent chapters.

Another aspect to use essential oils properly is to recognize that not all that is natural is harmful. The people who make this mistake do not realize that some plants (e.g. poison oak and poison ivy) can be harmful to people, and certain plants can be deadly if ingested (e.g. the yew plant). A variety of substances with animal origin are deadly as well, similar to the venom of a few snake species.

Essential oils from poisonous plants are primarily produced for chemists working in the field, however occasionally, they can be purchased by people who are not companies that are not reputable. In this book, harmful essential oils are not discussed. For those who are just beginning you should stick to essential oils that have been tested as safe such as lavender tea tree oil and rose instead of trying to try out new types.

Furthermore, a person could be sensitive to a harmless organic substance e.g. the nuts and strawberries. For those who suffer from a variety of allergies are generally advised to stay clear of essential oils, not just the ones that are generally safe, such as lavender. Individuals with specific medical issues such as pregnancy and lactating women, people taking prescription drugs as well as those suffering from asthma and so on. should also talk to their physician before experimenting with essential oils.

The advice above is not to scare you , but simply to keep you sure. It is well-known that certain chemicals even though they are considered safe for most people may interact with certain medicines or cause physical conditions. For instance, the over-the-counter acne medicine salicylic acid is suitable for pregnant and not lactating, however it is is not suitable for other women.

For those who don't suffer from a variety of allergies or have particular medical issues essential oils are generally secure. However, it's advised to perform an allergy test prior to doing. For this, you need to apply only a small amount of essential oil onto your skin, preferring to do this in an "hidden" area of your body such as behind your ear. If there is no irritation within 24 hours, it implies that this essential oil is suitable for apply. If irritation is observed it is necessary to get the area removed immediately and the oil should not be used.

This advice is not intended to discourage or scare users to avoid using essential oils, but to protect you. The majority of people who aren't suffering from allergies can make use of essential oils in a safe manner, however the human body can be unpredictable. One person could be one of millions who has an allergy that is unique to. If this is the case, any benefit you may get through the use of essential oils will be wiped out.

The third factor in making use of essential oils properly is knowing the correct method of use based on the function. They can be utilized in three methods: applied topically, inhaled for scent, or ingestion. The three methods will be described more in detail in subsequent chapters.

Chapter 5: Weight Loss Essential Oils Recipes

Mixing essential oils together is a fantastic opportunity to play by blending your favorite scents while reaping amazing healing benefits from each of the substances. There are numerous recipes that mix oils to create desired effects for physical and emotional well-being These recipes to lose weight will be an excellent introduction to reducing your appetite and removing undesirable fat.

Cellulite Blasting Rub:

To make this recipe, you'll require mixing 2 drops of oil from ginger, 2 drops peppermint oils, 2 drops Cypress oil, five drops of rosemary, and 10 of grapefruit. Mix them with the carrier oil like almond oil and apply it to the body parts that you would like to rid yourself of cellulite.

Massage Oil for Banishing fat:

To make this oil Mix one quarter cup of olive oil pure along with five drops Cypress oil and 5 drops lemon and five grapefruit. Apply this oil to your skin.

A Healthful Bath to Rejuvenate:

Infuse five drops of oil from lemon, five drops sandalwood five of orange grapefruit, and ginger to your hot bath to experience an energizing, relaxing experience.

Diffusion to Appetite Inhibiting Effects:

To curb your appetite and reduce weight to reduce appetite and shed weight, mix 40 drops essential oils of mandarin with 20 of lemon oil 12 drops peppermint, and 12 drops ginger oils. After you've got this mixture prepared you can place it into your diffuser, or just breathe in the aroma to lessen your appetite.

A soak to boost your metabolism

To make this bath recipe make sure to fill the tub with warm water. Add some tablespoons of almond oil as well as the grapefruit oil, eight drops and 10 drops of each of rosemary and cypress oils.

A Solution to Banishing cravings:

To make this diet, blend half 1 cup of olive oil extra virgin 75 drops of fennel oiland patchesouli oils 22 drops along with 35 drops Bergamot. Mix the ingredients together and then rub it on your abdomen to eliminate those annoying desire for unhealthy, fattening food items.

Chapter 6: Oils Essential for Arthritis Pain

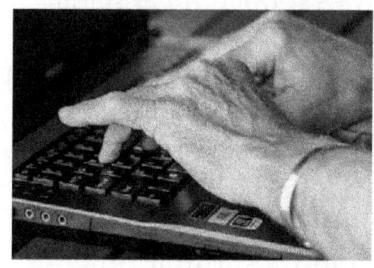

There are many who suffer from arthritis or Rheumatoid arthritis. There are some dietary restrictions that can help the joint swelling that cause pain, however, for those days when the weather is cold and your joints aren't letting up, there are handful of essential oils that you can apply to help:

Essential oils that are already are covered

Chamomile (Roman), Eucalyptus, Lavender, and Peppermint are all essential oils that possess anti-inflammatory properties that aid in relieving arthritis pain.

Additional essential oils

They are essential oils that will further aid in reducing the inflammation caused by arthritis and Rheumatism. The addition of these oils can assist in the treatment of pain caused by these ailments.

Black Pepper

(Piper nigrum) (Piper nigrum) is an essential oil which is highly recommended for instances of arthritis and rheumatism. It adds a healing warmth to a mixture that can ease discomfort and swelling.To be taken in small dosages.

Juniper

(Juniperus communis) It is an essential oil that helps to eliminate the toxin build-up which causes the pain of rheumatoid and also help be used to prevent arthritis.Not to be taken if pregnant or suffering from kidney disease.

Rosemary

(Rosmarius officinalis) It is a different oil that is often used in preparations and blends for rheumatism. Not advised for those suffering from hypertension or epilepsy. Avoid if you are pregnant.

Arthritis Salve

1 cup Sweet Almond or Apricot Kernel oil

1/8-cup Beeswax Beads

1/5 tsp peppermint EO

1/5 Drops Juniper EO

15 Drops Black Pepper EO

10 Drops of Clove oil

* In a double-boiler, put the oil and beeswax in a double boiler for melting the wax.

Mix the essential oils

* Pour the hot oil into a tightly-sealed container

* If you are sure that the mix is functional enough to stir, add all the oils essential to your diet.

Rub the joints to ease discomfort.

Arthritis Soak

1 Cup Epsom Salts

12 Cup Sea salt

1/4 Cup baking Soda

1/4 Cup Borax (It's a natural mineral)

1 Ounce Sweet Almond, or Apricot Kernel

1/5 tsp of Roman Chamomile EO

1/5 tsp peppermint EO

15 Drops Geranium Oil

5 Drops Clove 5 Drops Clove

You use a lesser quantity of the carrier oil as you also use minerals and salts to dilute essential oils.

Mix the oils, then put aside.

Mix all dry ingredients, and then set aside.

Add the oils slowly to dry ingredients, mixing it thoroughly.

* Place the contents in a sealed container for the night.

The mineral bath can be added in 1/8 Cup increments into warm water.

Mix well into the bath water, then allow to soak.

* You can also pour the mix in 1/8 cup measurements into the bowl of hot water and use it to make compress.

Arthritis Soak II

1 Cup Epsom Salts

12 Cup Sea salt

1/4 Cup baking Soda

1/4 Cup Borax (It's a natural mineral)

1 Ounce Sweet Almond, or Apricot Kernel

1/5 tsp of Roman Chamomile EO

1/5 tsp Juniper EO

15 Drops Helichrysum EO

5 Drops Clove 5 Drops Clove

It is recommended to use a lower quantity of the carrier oil as you also use minerals and salts to reduce the essential oils.

Mix the oils together and put aside.

Mix all dry ingredients, and then set aside.

Add the oils slowly into the dry ingredient, mixing thoroughly.

* Place the contents in a sealed container for the night.

• Add mineral baths in 14 Cup increments into warm water.

Mix well into the bath water. Let it take a bath and.

* You can also pour the mix in 1/8 cup measurements into an unheated bowl and use it to make compress.

Arthritis Ointment

4 ounces non-petroleum jelly

1/5 TSP Eucalyptus EO

10 Drops Lavender EO

10 Drops Juniper EO

15 Drops Rosemary Drops

10 Drops Black Pepper EO

* Heat the jelly gently until it melts in the double boiler.

* Place the contents in a covered container that is tightly sealed.

Mix essential oils and include them once the jelly is warm

Ointment for Arthritis that is free of Rosemary

4 ounces non-petroleum jelly

1/5 tsp peppermint EO

10 Drops Geranium Essential Oil

Ten Drops Roman Chamomile EO

15 Drops Juniper EO

10 Drops Black Pepper EO

* Heat the jelly gently until it is melted in the double boiler.

* Place it in a covered container that is tightly sealed.

Mix essential oils and include them once the jelly is warm

Oil to relieve pain and arthritis

3 1/2 Ounces 3 1/2 Ounces of Sweet Almond and Apricot Kernel Oil

1/2 Ounce Cold-pressed Sesame Oil

1/5 TSP Eucalyptus EO

Ten Drops Roman Chamomile EO

10 Drops of Rosemary EO

10 Drops Black Pepper EO

Ten Drops of Clove Oil

Combine all oils in a bowl and mix thoroughly.

* Rub your fingers into the joints to reduce the swelling and ease pain.

Oil of Arthritis-Free Rosemary

3 1/2 Ounces 3 1/2 Ounces of Sweet Almond as well as Apricot Kernel Oil

12 Ounce Sesame Oil

1/5 tsp Lavender EO

1/5 tsp Juniper EO

15 drops Roman Chamomile EO

10 Drops Black Pepper EO

Blend all of the oil and mix thoroughly.

Rub the affected joints to reduce the swelling and relieve pain.

Chapter 7: Oil Pulling with Essential Oils

What's the oil pulling?

It's a low-cost simple, safe, and non-complicated process which can offer you many advantages, ranging from maintaining your mouth's health and free of harmful bacteria and toxic substances. It can also serve as a treatment and way to prevent illnesses, allowing you to live longer and healthier.

A few of its advantages are:

Whiter and brighter teeth

Healthier gums

Preventing bad breath

A boost in energy

Fewer migraine attacks

A clearer and more focused mind. concentration

Allergies are a common cause of allergic reactions.

Treatment for insomnia

Clearer sinuses

Menstrual cycles that are better controlled

Better skin health

Better lymphatic system

Lessened PMS symptoms

Essential oils that are the best to pull:

Peppermint. This is an excellent option if looking to boost your energy and also an increase in your mental and physical power. It's also beneficial to eliminate bad breath, as well as to ease any headaches you might be suffering from. If you have digestive problems, this could benefit you as well.

Orange. Have you experienced mood swings recently? Maybe you're in a perpetual low mood that you cannot manage to shake? This is the essential oil for you. It also aids in detoxification and stopping weight gain.

Grapefruit. On a diet? This essential aspect particularly will help you to curb your cravings and reducing your appetite. It can stop your from eating excessively and aid in losing weight. It's also a great option for those who are suffering from hangovers.

Lemon. This lemon is multi-purpose. It's fantastic to ease the symptoms of colds effectively and swiftly. It also provides a boost both in mood and focus. It can also assist you deal with stress and reduce it. For your body, it is excellent for cleansing and detoxification that will help you get rid of any toxins accumulation.

Oregano. The most common remedy for toothaches It is one of the top essential oils you can use for oil pulling. It also provides users with other advantages, including relief from throat soreness and asthma. It also assists in the prevention and treatment of parasites, as well as viral infections.

Rosemary. This essential oil is fantastic to boost your immunity and also decongesting the liver. If you've experienced soreness, pains, and aches it could aid in easing all that. It also improves circulation and treats Candida extremely effectively.

Chapter 8: The Essential Oil And Stress

Everyday we are confronted with stress as well as deadlines for work and pressures from our families and society. A lot of times we are under stress to the point where stress can become a normal aspect of our lives. Stress can affect different biological processes, including the managing weight as well as fatigue, anxiety and depression. Stress can cause thyroid and hormonal adrenal conditions.

Essential oils can help relieve stress.

Smell has the ability to significantly affect our mood, primarily due to the fact that smell is directly connected to our limbic system within our cortex (the central nervous system that is the emotional centre of our brain). This means that the sense of smell does not just affect our mood, but also other bodily processes that occur in our body. When we breathe in essential oils the molecules are channeled through receptors in the Olfactory system. The receptors transmit the information from compounds to our brains, leading to the sensation of smell. The olfactory bulbs being an element of the limbic system, captures information via its senses, and stores it as memories. This is the reason why you may smell a specific scent and instantly experience flashbacks to certain memories. Given that our limbic system can be involved in regulating high levels of stress, using essential oils can have psychological and physiological affects on our physical as well as emotional health. Below are a few essential oils that can be used for healing which are believed to help emotional and mental issues:

Lavender

Lavender oil is among the most widely used oil used for relieving anxiety and stress. The lavender plant is a source of linalyl as well as Linalool, which can cross the barrier between blood and brain, affecting the brain's activity in a matter of minutes. According to a study which took place in the year 2012 the smell of lavender oil will not only make you feel more relaxed, but makes you feel sharper.

Bergamot

Bergamot is known for its ability to stimulate the endocrine system, and aids in the creation of a feeling of peace and well-being. This aids in reducing stress levels. Add about six drops of the oil bergamot into your bath and then take a bath to relax. It is also possible to put five drops of oil from bergamot into the steaming water in a bowl , then put a towel between your head and in the bowl to release the steam then inhale it for a while.

Frankincense

Frankincense is a warm, exotic scent that helps people feel peace and calm. Take a whiff of this essential oil each whenever you feel like things are out of hand; it can do a decent job of relaxing you.

Ylang Ylang

The essential oil can be helpful in helping you focus your thoughts and gives you an increased sense of well-being and tranquility. Inhaling the scent of ylang ylang can make you feel better.

Vanilla

The vanilla's scent alone will make you feel comfortable. Many aromatherapists believe that vanilla has the closest aroma and flavor that mothers milk. Vanilla helps make you feel calm and improves mental clarity. Put vanilla in a diffuser and enjoy the amazing aroma.

Tangerine

Tangerine is quite effective in enabling you overcome depression.

Lemon

Lemon is vital because it can provide a relaxing, comforting, and energizing sensation when it is inhaled.

Chamomile

Chamomile is also very efficient as a sedative as well as relaxing aid.

Chapter 9: The Essential Oils that Are Safe for Children

At a certain point children become more tolerant to things like medication and essential oils that are strong. From the time they are born to early adulthood they're delicate little creatures.

In the case of supplements and vitamins, certain doses and kinds of oils essential to life are suitable for children.

It's not an issue you want to put off to guesswork. This is why it is the goal in this section to determine the essential oils that are safe, and in what amounts.

Colds: Mix 2 tablespoons vegetable oils with 2 drops Tea Tree, 1 drop of Lemon* along with 1 drop Ross Otto essential oils. Massage this blend onto the chest and neck. (you could also try substituting Cedarwood*, Rosemary** Rose, Sandalwood or Thyme)

Colic: For children who suffer from colic, mix 2 tablespoons of almond oils, just one drop Roman Chamomile, 1 drop of Lavender and one drop Geranium. Apply this mixture to the stomach and return. It's a good idea to use warm (but still not too hot) water is also beneficial when placed on the stomach. It can also be used Bergamot* Ginger, Mandarin*, Marjoram, Rosemary or Ylang-Ylang.

Constipation: Dilute one of the Ginger, Mandarin*, Orange* or Rosemaryessential oils and apply them to the abdomen and feet.

Cradle Cap: Mix 2 tablespoons Almond Oil with 1 drop of Lemon* and 1 drop of Geranium (or with 1 drop of Cedarwood** and 1 drop of Sandalwood). Place a small amount on your baby's scalp.

The Croup Dilute Marjoram, Rosewood, Sandalwood or Thyme and gently massage your baby. It is also possible to use them as a diffuser. Fresh air and cold temperatures could also be helpful, as that the baby is properly wrapped.

Diaper Rash Mix 1 drop Lavender with 1 drop Roman Chamomile with vegetable oil and apply.

Digestion dilute Lemon* , or Orangeessential oils then massage these oils into your feet and stomach.

Dry Skin Dry Skin Rosewood as well as Sandalwood essential oils, and then apply the oil to your affected area.

Earaches: dilute and apply Lavender as well as tea Tree, Roman Chamomile, and Sweet Thyme. Put a drop of mixture on the cotton ball. Rub the cotton ball gently across the child's ear as well as on the ear's Vitaflex Points ***.

Fevers: Dilute the essential lavender oil by mixing vegetable oil. Massage the child or baby on the side of their neck on their feet, or behind their ears. (You may also apply peppermint, however if you are using it, make sure to diffuse it.)

Flu: Mix a drop from Cypress, Lemon*, and Tea Tree essential oils in bath gel, and then use them in the bath of your baby.

Hiccups: Diffuse Mandarin* essential oil.

The remedy for jaundice is to dilute the Geranium Citrus* and Lime* Mandarin* as well as Rosemary**, and apply it to the liver as well as on the Vita Flex Points of the liver. ***.

Refluxes: Mix then apply Lavender, Roman chamomile, Rose Otto or sandalwood.

Teeth Grinding The best way to prevent this is to gently rub Lavender on the soles of their feet.

Tonsillitis: Dilute one of Ginger, Lavender, Lemon*, Tea Tree, or Roman Chamomile, and apply it to the skin underneath the tonsils.

Thrush: Mix two tablespoons Garlic Oil with 8 drops Lavender and 8 drops Tea

Tree, and 1 milliliter of Vitamin E oil. Apply it directly to the nipples prior to nursing, and directly in the mouth of your baby with a finger that is clean.

*These oils are photosensativeand should be always dilute. To avoid skin rash or a pigmentation of the skin, avoid using citrus oils in direct sunlight.

These oils should not be applied undiluted to babies and children.

*Vita Flex Points are pressure points that are located on your feet. Each one corresponds to a area that is part of you. To use these points correctly simply press then roll and release in an upward motion to cover the correct point. Essential oils will be absorbed through the skin into capillaries and the bloodstream, delivering its healing qualities to their desired area within the human body.

Premature Babies

Since babies born prematurely have extremely thin skin, and are sensitive to a variety of products and chemicals It is recommended to stay clear of applying essential oils in a unified way until they've had the chance to develop more resilience to the chemicals.

Cosmetic Uses

Essential oils are used in cosmetics for hundreds of years. They are safe and natural than the majority of products on the market. in addition, they revitalize and improve the health of your hair, skin and nails while delivering the results you want immediately and are a sustainable method of personal care.

Hair Care

Essential oils are wonderful for hair. It doesn't matter whether you suffer from dry hair, lice, dandruff or hair that is oily, there's an essential oil appropriate for your needs. There are oils that, if used correctly, can aid in the loss of hair and early hair loss.

To avoid dandruff For instance make a mixture of five drops of Lemon oil 2 drops Lavender oil 1 drop of Rosemary along with 2 drops peppermint oil in 2 tablespoons of an oil carrier (I prefer coconut oil to treat hair problems). Massage the mixture onto your scalp, and allow it to rest for 10 minutes before washing it off. Then, you are able to simply shampoo your hair like you would normally.

It is also possible to use Tea Tree and Manuka oil in dandruff preventative mixtures.

To prevent hair loss For hair loss prevention, mix 3 drops Rosemary oil with 3 drops Cedarwood along with 3 drops Lavender together with 2 ounces carrier oil (like coconut oil) into the container. Massage the mix into hair, and allow it to remain on for upto an hour. Apply this treatment at least once or twice per week. You can also put 1 or 2 drops of Rosemary or Carrot oil on your hair brush prior to brushing to encourage hair growth if your hair is starting to thin.

Other oils that can help prevent hair loss include Bay oil, lemon oil and Mustard oil, as well as Peppermint oil.

To revive dry hair, you can make an oil conditioner that is hot (really that's warm oil conditioner because scalding oils can cause dangersome burns and be able to harm the hair). To make this happen mix 15 drops Rosewood with 5 drops of Sandalwood five drops of Geranium and five drops Lavender as well as 4 tablespoons carrier oil (like coconut oil). Put this mixture into the bag of a small plastic container and then soak it in a the temperature of a hot cup for up to one minute. When it's warm, rub the mixture into hair and allow it to rest (wrapped in an apron) for 20 minutes prior to washing it off.

You can also apply Mustard oil to revive your hair, and Lemongrass oil to help strengthen it in the event that it's dry and fragile.

To treat oily hair, mix 9 drops of Ylang Ylang, 9 drops of lime, and 9 drops Rosemary along with 2 tablespoons carrier oil. Massage the mixture on your head , then rinse it off in two minutes. It is recommended to do this at least three times per week.

Head lice can be prevented from recurring with a mixture of 3 drops Thyme oil Lavender oil, and three drops of Geranium in 10 drops of carrier oil (Sweet Almond oil works well to do this). Massage this mixture into your scalp and then cover the head using a shower cap. Allow this to sit for approximately 30 minutes prior to shampooing as normal.

Nail Care

Your nails go through many strains during the day, especially when you employ traditional cleaning products or perform any manual work. Women shell out lots of money to make their nails look better in salons, however many of the manicures we buy cause our nails to be dry broken, cracked, and brittle.

To help strengthen your nails (especially during manicures) Mix 10 drops of Frankincense Oil, 10 drops Myrrh oil along with 10 drops Lemon oil. Add two tablespoons Vitamin E oil (you can purchase Vitamin E oil as gel caps, or as liquid. If you are unable to locate the liquid, gel caps work when you crush the coating of rubber and squeeze the oil out. This isn't easy and time-consuming, however you should try to find the liquid version.)

Mix all the ingredients and keep the mixture in an opaque transparent glass bottle (the bottle that the essential oils is in will suffice). Apply the mixture to your cuticles and allow it to soak in between manicures, or every other week if you don't usually do your nails.

Skin Care

The benefits that are attributed to using essential oils for your skin can be extensive. In actual fact, when you take a look, the majority of the advertising for products for skincare (and products for hair care, in particular) is focused on the ingredients that the product is made of (ie products that are infused with Lemon or peppermint.)

This is due to the fact that in many instances, the plant-based infusions are where the majority of the rejuvenating and healing properties originate from (Ha. Stem. We did what?)

All-Natural Lotion

For a pure lotion make a mixture of 10 drops Myrrh with fifteen drops Geranium along with 5 drops Ylang-Ylang in an oil carrier (coconut oil is a great choice).

All-Natural Sunscreen

To protect yourself naturally from harmful UV rays, blend 5 drops Myrrh oil and 5 drops of carrot oil and 10 drops of carrier oil (Sweet Almond oil or Aloe Vera can be used in this case) to make a sunscreen that has 40 SPF.

to reduce wrinkles

Blend 5 drops Sandalwood oil with four drops Geranium oil 3 drops Lavender oil, and six drops of Frankincense in an oil carrier (like coconut oil). Massage this mixture into your skin every day, but make sure you keep it away from your eyes.

To Reduce Stretchmarks

This is a great option in case you've recently shed weight or have recently become pregnant. It also helps in preventing stretchmarks in your pregnancy. Blend 5 drops Frankincense oil five drops Myrrh oil 5 drops of Coriander oil, and 5 drops of Lavender together with

5 drops an oil carrier (like coconut oil). Massage this mixture onto your stretchmarks at least twice every day.

Skin Toner

To tone your skin blend 8 ounces of pure water with 2 drops Lavender oil and 2 drops Palmarosa oil two drops Rosewood. A cotton ball is dipped in the toner, and apply it to your face, gently upward strokes. Place the mixture in a bottle of water and shake it prior to each application.

Facial Scrub

For a clean and clear complexion Apply 3 drops of Lemon oil three drops Tea Tree oil, and 3 drops of Sweet Orange oil to the affected region. It is best to make use of a clean cotton ball for this.

To create a facial scrub we suggest making a mixture of 1/4 cup yogurt plain, 1/4 cup of cornmeal five drops Patchouli Oil, five drops Grapefruit oil, and 4 drops Lavender oil. The mix can be stored at room temperature for up to three days.

to minimize the appearance of Scars

There are many essential oils that can be helpful in decreasing signs of scar tissue. One reason for this is the fact that many oils aid in cellular renewal and growth. Of these oils that are most effective, they include Bergamot oil Chamomile oil Fennel oil Galbanum oil Helicrysum oil Hyssop oil and Jasmine oils. Manuka oil and Neroli oil.

To Tighten Skin

To increase and tighten the elasticity of your skin you can use the Geranium oil and Peppermint oil.

Deodorants, perfumes and breath Fresheners

If there's one thing that should be emphasized on, it's this: fragrances and colognes aren't essential oils. They do not possess the same therapeutic properties , and they'll always be some chemical smell to them due to the fact that they are made in high-pressure environments at extreme temperatures, effectively dissolving the chemical properties of essential oils.

The companies do this to make them more efficient and then sell them at a lower cost. This alters the chemical composition of the oil however, and produce an inferior product that could even contain toxins, based on the oil used and the mixture it was used with other chemicals.

To make your own fragrance that is all natural or deodorizer Follow these steps:

Perfumes

Blend 25 drops from Lavender, Patchouli oil, Sandalwood as well as Geranium together with one ounce vodka that is good quality (it must at least be triple or twice distilled). Let the mixture sit for about two weeks prior to using it. Spray using a diffuser spray it (you can buy them at the dollar shop).

Deodorants

Create your own deodorant with any of Benzoin, Citronella, Coriander, Cypress, Eucalyptus, Geranium, Manuka, Myrtle, Neroli, or Rose Geranium. Mix 5 drops of the mixture with 2 ounces Coconut oil and store it in a container that is sealed within the fridge.

It's not an antiperspirant. It's an anti-odorant. It is best to use it during exercise which is when you're supposed to eliminate all your toxic substances. This allows you to continue sweating and flush out the toxins, without causing a stink in the space. Antiperspirants aren't all as beneficial to your health and are best employed only in situations where you do not want pits on your shirt...like in the workplace or out on dates. Avoid them while exercising.

You can also put Geranium oil or lemon oil on cotton balls, then place them inside your shoes for a freshener the air after a long run.

Remedy for Bad Breath

Although this solution is, obviously, not by any meant to substitute cleaning your teeth with toothpaste, it is possible to make use of it as a quick fix to fresh breath problems. Combine two drops Cinnamon essential oil with two tablespoons Coconut oil. Then, you can swish the mixture around your mouth for anywhere between 1 to 15 minutes before pulling it into and down your teeth.

This method is a twist on the well-known method known as Oil Pulling. This method will not only improve your breath, it can also help with headaches, improve your teeth's whiteness as well as help in the elimination of gingivitis and even aid those who suffer from TMJ.

Make sure that you throw your mixture in the garbage bin to avoid ingesting essential oils. Ingestion of essential oils isn't recommended. The poisons you've gotten out of your mouth are only going to re-enter your body, negating the entire purpose.

Chapter 10: Increasing Market The Rise Of Essential Oils

If essential oils are a bit questionable scientifically, and there's a some healthy debate about their uses how come they are everywhere? This is an amazing and thought-provoking question I asked you to consider and here's the quick answer.

Essential oils are extremely affordable and aren't discredited. In spite of not discrediting essential oils, and lacking the evidence behind their claims to show they're not effective medical professionals aren't sure about even removing these oils. What it does provide however is the reality of the reason they're not widely marketed.

Money is the answer.

The medical industry is infected and awash with money and the influence of pharmaceutical corporations, which are among of the biggest and frightening industries around the globe. They have control over every aspect of what occurs. From the congress to the tiny clinics that are in the middle of the desert.

A donation or the support of a pharmaceutical firm can transform everything, and there's one thing they are concerned about, and that's making the possibility of making a profit. If your company sells drugs which make people feel better or relieves the symptoms of illness it's an industry that is dying. If you're one of one of the most lucrative and exclusive industry in the world , and it is also self-terminating Are you truly concerned about curing and helping others or are you just looking to make making money?

The answer lies in money, and that's no the case with conspiracy theories. The evidence is overwhelming that pharmaceutical firms are more interested in making money rather than providing you with a medication which will cure you of your disease.

When a challenge is held against ibuprofen, which is made in the in the middle of nowhere at a cost of almost nothing pharmaceutical companies are will be pushing for the medical profession to deny it and maintain a healthy skeptical views regarding it. Therefore, if doctors did come out and declare that essential oils are safe and effective in a significant way, they could lose huge amounts of money supporting their research, practice and even their lives.

You'll find that nearly everyone has been exposed to essential oils, and there are testimonies everywhere claiming that essential oils actually assisted them, and they're not those who are selling the product to anyone else. If something is effective and being criticized by the top dogs of society, it's going to last and that's exactly the way essential oils have accomplished for hundreds of years.

There's no way to be able to eliminate them since they work. If they weren't working they would be slammed and discarded years ago, yet they've endured.

The market has exploded again. There are people who will purchase them to assist them deal with ailments that they don't want to invest forty dollars to fix. Consider how much sleep aids or drops to treat sore throats cost. Take note of the amount you spend on them annually and the cost. In a fraction of the amount you've paid for cold medicines you could be purchasing just one container of oils that will not be more expensive than what the amount you're spending. That's the reason why the market has endured.

With a rapidly growing market at the cost that essential oils are priced it's worth talking to an official. Find someone who you can believe in and speak with them the next time you're suffering from an aching throat or sleepless night.

They offer remedies and cures that can help you overcome all the things that could cause harm to you. The bottom line is that I believe this is the final test as to whether something is legitimate or not.

Take a look around and save cash on cold medicines this winter and test some essential oils to determine whether they're as good as they're made for. If they don't work well, then, you're out a tiny amount of money. However, I can assure you that they'll work for you.

"The Power of Nature: Dangers and Security

We now know what essential oils are and where they're derived from, how they're utilized and the reason why they've lasted for the past ten years and beyond, I think it's high time to address something that will undoubtedly pop in the course of researching essential oils. It's the warning.

Before we get any further than this I want to be sure that you are aware of rules and standards which will protect yourself from anything you're fearful of. They're not going bottle pure nightshade or acid and then sell it to the public.

But since these are all organic, natural substances and when used at their maximum potency they can be extremely damaging to you. It is therefore important to understand the risks and issues that may arise in the event of abuse of essential oils or make the wrong connections.

The entire chapter is directed at those who want to go organic and are looking to buy at a local apothecary is set up by someone in the hopes of starting an organization. Simple things can turn dangerous and it's essential to show respect of the things nature is capable of.

The first thing you'll want to understand is that diluting is the solution to any issue that is associated from the strength in essential oils. The

Higher the purity, more dangerous the product will be for the person. Therefore, before buying an extract of cinnamon from a man with a beard that is long and a flannel-tshirt Make sure the seller has declared purity and has done his research about the product. You don't want to burn your skin. If an essential oil is excessively powerful for the body, it can cause serious issues, particularly on sensitive areas such as your mouth or eyes. Essential oils can be utilized for aromatherapy or consumption to ease the symptoms of congestion and pain.

Another time that you shouldn't be using essential oils is when you're pregnant. Essential oils are extremely concentrated quantities of plant essences which are the scent of plants. If you're knowledgeable about pregnant women, then you'll be able to understand precisely where I'm coming from with this. Essential oils have a strong scent and if you're trying to get a pregnant woman to want to kill you, or exile them from your life forever Bring something smoky around. All in all, I'd suggest against using essential oils if you're pregnant, are planning to be pregnant, or have a pregnant woman near you. It's all common sense in this one.

If you're planning to take the route of purchasing from an apothecary in your area then you must do the necessary research about what type of shop you'll be purchasing from. One of the main factors be looking for is quality and the product that you're getting.

It is important to purchase from stores that offer suppliers that are 100 100% organic. The reason behind this is that there are hazardous and harmful pesticides that are utilized to ensure that plants and crops are free from pests that destroy the crops. If you're not using oils that are controlled and completely natural and safe, the risk of having poisons absorbed into your body, breathed in, or even in your mouth. The risk is enough to be a possibility. Be aware to take care of yourself and recognize that you're putting toxic substances on your body. One of the best ways to tell whether the local company whom you're dealing with legitimate request an overview or request evidence that they're working with secure business practices.

It is very easy to end up poisoning yourself if not mindful when it comes to controlling essential oils. They are extremely concentrated, powerful substances that have been diluted to ensure your protection and safety. When you consume excessive amounts of an essence, you can be causing serious damage for your health. If something isn't working, the remedy is not to continue taking more or increasing the dose without consulting an expert who can provide advice on the issue first.

Use your brain, and ensure it is secure. Essential oils are essential to stay healthy and not to harm yourself. Remember that.

Chapter 11: Essential Oils: All About

The use of essential oils goes from the beginning of time. Egyptians employed them in their embalming process as being used in their cosmetics as well as the burning of incense which included essential oils.They made use of aromatic herbs for medicinal, religious and aromatherapy purposes.They were also used over the years for their healing properties in traditional medicine since the beginning of time, and much of it remains in use similar to how we use them today.

"essential oils" is a term that comes from "essential oils" originates from "quintessential oil."This comes from the Aristotelian concept that matter was made up of four elements: water, fire and air.The vital force or the spirit that a plant has was believed as the 5th element, or quintessence.During it's process evaporation and distillation was believed to be when "spirits" were taken away from plants. Nowadays, we are aware the essential oils to be physical and comprise an intricate mix of chemicals.

Essential Oils are a form of concentrated hydrophobic liquids that are a source of aroma compounds from plants they're obtained from by various means that involve extraction.Other terms that the essential oils can be referred to as are volatile oil, ethereal oils the word aetherola, as well as plainly"oil from" the plant from which was extracted from.Oils are called essential due to their smell of the plant they originate from.Essential oils are not necessary to health, however they are often used for medicinal uses, particularly when they are used in conjunction with alternative therapies.

Nowadays, distillation is the most popular method for gathering essential oil since it is simple to separate liquid water.During the process the plants are put within the still, and then placed in the grid. The still is then shut shut. Depending on the process of distillation water or steam is passed through the plant material, taking out the volatile constituents. These ascend and pass through a pipe connecting them that leads it into the condenser. The condenser cools the vapor to the liquid form. There is a storage container beneath the condenser to collect the liquid. The essential oils and water are not compatible, and essential oils are taken at the top of the container using siphoning method. Sometimes essential oils weigh more than water, in which situation, and are taken out of below the collector. Described below is a brief overview of different methods.

Water Distillation:

This is a method of extraction that involves materials from plants are brought in direct contact with water. This method is typically employed with orange and flowers blossoms since steam pressure causes them to become clumped together, which makes it hard for steam to move through.

Steam and Water:

This process is used in conjunction with leaf and herb materials. the water is kept below the plant material throughout this procedure. The steam is pumped out from the main still in indirect ways.

Steam Distillation:

It is by far the most frequently employed method of extraction. The steam gets injected the cylinder at a greater temperature and pressure than the other two methods.

Percolation:

It is the most up-to-date method, it's like steam distillation, but instead of steam flowing from the bottom of the still it is pushed through the top.This type of extraction allows more efficient distillation time.It works well for extraction essential oils out of difficult materials like wood.

Expression (Cold Press):

This technique is typically employed in the collection of essential oils of citrus. The peels are usually pressed by mechanical machines to extract oil essentials from peels.

Below are some of the most important oils as well as their advantages and applications

Olive Essential Oil

• Good for heart health

* Rich in monounsaturated fatty acids

* Olive oil could lower your risk of developing heart disease through lowering cholesterol

Argan Oil

Argan oil is served as a beauty treatment for centuries.

This oil is ideal to multi-task.

* Aids in brittle nails.

* Great to apply to dry and rough skin

Rosehip Oil

* A powerful exfoliant

* Rich in vitamin E

* Helps to improve the appearance and brightness of your skin.

* Rosehip is a rich source of essential fatty acids that can help with dry skin conditions like Psoriasis and eczema.

Lavender Oil

* For stress relief

The scent of lavender can help lower stress hormones in your blood.

* It can help you sleep or rest in the night (try adding oil to your pillow)

* Excellent for skin that is dry and scaly.

Manuka Oil

* Has anti-fungal properties

* Can aid in healing scrapes and cuts.

Peppermint Oil

* May help relieve symptoms of irritable bowel syndrome.

* It can be taken in.

Mix a small amount of water to ease the symptoms of indigestion.

Lemon Essential Oil

Lemons are a great source of properties that reduce stress. They are incorporated into the oil

Spray lemons to aid in relaxing after a an exhausting day at work

* Grate lemon peels and fill the bottle to half-way with rinds. Fill the remaining portion with oil. Let it rest on the window sill for a couple of days. to keep you in a relaxed state through the smell of

Oil of Oregano

* is one of the most potent antibiotics found in nature.

* Effective in eliminating bacteria.

* Helps the immune system combat fungi parasites, and viruses

* Containing the compound Carvacrolthat has been proven to break the membrane's outer layer that assists to guard against bacteria through invading the immune system.

The safe use of essential oils:

Be sure to know how to apply the specific essential oil you are planning to use. They aren't all applied or used in the identical manner.Taking these steps will allow you to avoid any severe negative side negative effects.

Your risk will be low If you utilize essential oils responsible and safe manner. Essential oils sold to be used in professional or household use are usually safe.If you adhere to the fundamental guidelines and guidelines there should be no problems making use of essential oils.You might experience a slight skin irritation , but nothing risky.

The guidelines to follow

Always use pure essential oils. There is a greater possibility of suffering from negative side effects with adulterated products and it is crucial to select only pure essential oils.

Diluting other oils

Certain essential oils, such as citrus-based oils can cause irritation to the skin in the event that they are not first dilute by a carrier oil like olive oil. Any oils which contain cinnamaldehyde, eugenol such as citronella, citrus or cinnamon need to be dilute prior to application on the skin.

Methods of applying essential oils:

Essential oils can be applied through ingestion or diffuse them inhaling or directly on the skin. Every method of application is a risky one that needs to be taken care of.

1) Skin application

Avoid applying oil to skin that has been damaged since the wound or open area can absorb more oils that usual and could lead you to take in dangerous amounts in essential oils. Try not to apply too many essential oils on your skin because this can cause irritation to your skin.

Essential oils that can cause irritation to skin include: Bay, Tagetes, Thyme, Oregano, Clove Bud, Lemongrass, Cinnamon bark and Cumin

2) Diffusion

It is a method of dispersing essential oils in the air to ensure that the aroma of the oils fills the room with the pure scent of essential oils. This method of application may be accomplished by the use of a nebulizer, or making use of incense. Other kinds of diffusion techniques are steam, simple diffusion candles, lamp rings, candle and the terracotta diffusers. The first recorded usage of this method was done by the Andalusian doctor, chemist and pharmacistIbn al-Baitar (1188-1248).

3)Internal ingestion

Essential oils are not able to be consumed internally, therefore it is crucial to ensure that you follow the guidelines to take essential oils internally.Some examples are lemon, lavender, and peppermint oils.

4)Inhaling

There's no reason to be concerned when taking essential oils into an enclosed space; but the correct guidelines should be adhered to.

Chapter 12: Essential Oils For Sleep Disorders & Tranquility

In our current state it is difficult to get the recommended five to six hours sleep. Even if those hours are devoted to sleeping, the majority of people don't get enough sleep during this time. The sleep they get is interrupted because of the stress and numerous health issues. Many people struggle to get between three and four hours of uninterrupted sleep. In the absence of adequate sleep, they don't feel healthy and energetic on the following day. They are prescribed medicines to help improve their condition and to get better sleep in the evening. The medications may ameliorate the condition, however they will not offer an end-to-end solution. The adverse effects of these medications are higher than the advantages. However, if you are using essential oils, you'll certainly feel better.

Essential oils include Roman oils of chamomile, valerian lavendar oil, bergamot oil cementwood oil Sweet marjoram oil clary sage oil, orange oil, and ylang-ylang oil are thought to be the best for sleep. Essential oils are used for insomnia and sleeping disorders.

Essential oil recipes for sleep problems and peace

1. Sleep well and get a good night's sleep.

The essential oil of lavender can bring your nervous system into the state of relaxation. The essential oil of valerian can help you sleep faster. It also helps to prolong your sleep. The oil of cedarwood is used to reduce the motor activity. It's also thought to be beneficial to extend your sleep. For a blend that works for any type of sleep disorders, make a mixture of the oils of lavender, cedarwood along with valerian oil. It is necessary to create the mixture using five drops of lavender oil and 2 drops cedarwood oils and three drops of valerian oil. Anyone suffering from sleep issues can make use of this blend to sleep quickly and remain at rest for an extended period. This blend can increase the quality and amount of sleep you get. Additionally, you will be refreshed and rejuvenated each morning. If you're having trouble sleeping it is possible to include a few drops of Roman chamomile oil into this mixture to help improve your state.

2. Doze

If you're having trouble getting to sleep due to work or stress, or muscle strain, you could utilize this blend to ease your mind and prepare your body for a peaceful sleep. It will let you sleep quickly. For making this blend, you'll require 3 drops of vetiver oils 4 drops orange oil, and 4 drops lavender oil and thirty milliliters of grapeseed oil.

3. Tranquility

If you're looking to get a good night's sleep You can include a few drops of this mix to your bath. A bath before going to bed can offer an improved result. This blend also helps to alleviate the effects of exercise on muscle discomfort. If you suffer from dry skin, make use of this mixture to help improve the condition of your skin. To create this blend, you'll require 3 drops of marjoram oil, three drops of oil from yarrow two drops of Geranium oil along with 20ml of bubbles.

Essential oils for insect bites and Repellent Spray

A bite from an insect can be extremely painful. In some instances insects bites can be dangerous. They can cause discomfort and swelling, as well as pain and itching. It is possible to use medicines to treat the problem and stop the spread of the disease. However, you can't take these medicines without having a prescription. The process can be long and can make the condition more severe. However, you can make essential oils to ease the symptoms and prevent the spread of illness.

Essential oils blend recipes to treat insect bites

1. To treat an insect bite

Essential oils can be used in blends to help reduce the symptoms that result from bites by insects. To make this blend, you'll require 10 drops Roman Chamomile oil, 5 drops peppermint oil and 12 drops lavender oil and 6 drops of oil from lemon.

2. Insect repellent spray

If you're plagued by a lot bugs in your yard and have trouble controlling them, try using essential oil blends to limit their spread and prevent their appearance. The blend will not harm the plants. It also emits pleasant scent that is not associated when you use the chemicals that are commonly used to kill insects that are in your garden. To make this blend you'll need twelve drops of rosemary oil. You will also need 10 drops peppermint oil and 8 drops of clove oil as well as 12 drops Thyme oil. These essential oils are believed to be effective in killing insects. However, they aren't dangerous to human beings. Spray this blend onto your soil in order to eliminate insects or to stop their appearance.

3. Bug repellent

Bugs are a frequent household issue. A lot of people suffer from bugs living in their homes. They have a variety of techniques to rid themselves of bugs for good. However, many don't offer an end-to-end solution. Even if people get relief for a short time but they don't get the same result for a long time. The bugs continue to come. If you're among the people who suffer from this, look into essential oils. It's a simple and easy method, but it will give you the best results. To create this blend, you'll require seven drops of lavender oil. 12 drops lemongrass oils, 10 Geranium oils and 8 drops peppermint oils.

4. For the purpose of preventing bacteria

If you are looking to eliminate the germs in your home and improve the cleanliness of your home and make it more hygiene-friendly, you might have spend some money on cleaning products every month. Additionally, these strategies may not be suitable for your pet or the children you have. If you're seeking a secure and a long-lasting solution you can try essential oils. To make this blend, you'll require the equivalent of 30 drops clove oil as well as 25, drops lemon oil five drops of eucalyptus oil 10-drops of the oil cinnamon and three drops of the rosemary oil. The blend is a great way to shield your home from bacteria and eliminate them.

Essential oils offer numerous advantages. It is easy to put one drop of lavender oil and place it on an unbleached cotton ball and apply it to your skin directly to avoid mosquitoes. If you're looking to add humidity to your home, just add 9 drops of Tea tree oils. You can also make use of essential oils for an air freshener. You can choose any essential oil of your choice. A couple of drops of oil can revive the air and the environment. Furthermore, these oils are safe and do not cause allergies. Even if you suffer from breathing issues and are sensitive to the air freshener, it is possible to use essential oils. They will not bother you in any way. All you have to do is select the appropriate essential oil and combination to achieve the desired outcome.

Chapter 13: Benefits Of Essential Oils

Essential oils offer a variety of advantages and we're going to take a look at a few of them.

Are able to penetrate your skin immediately

One of the advantages from essential oils they can be absorbed by your skin cell membranes quickly. It takes only a few minutes for them to spread through your tissues and blood. These oils are able to pass through the blood-brain barrier to gain access to the amygdale and other limbic regions of the brain. These are the brain regions that are responsible for managing our mood as well as our beliefs and emotions. That means that essential oils can be capable of transforming these three to help us deal with stress, anger , and other emotions that we may be confronted with.

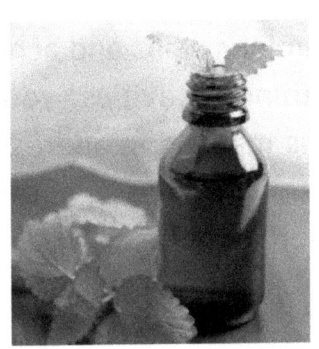

They are oxygen-rich and have properties

Essential oils contain oxygen molecules. They are able to transport oxygen to cells within our bodies that are deficient of oxygen, and also to cells that require nutrition too. Cells in our bodies require oxygen so that they are in a position to function effectively and essential oils assist in this.

They ease joint and muscle pain.

If you're suffering from pain in your muscles or joints, essential oils may be the best solution. It is possible that you experience minor pains and aches because of the routine activities you do, and essential oils may aid in addressing this. If you mix them with massage, then you will see even more benefits.

They're rich in antioxidants.

Essential oils are known for their high concentration of antioxidants that aid the body. Antioxidants help strengthen your body's systems. They help the body stop the negative effects that lifestyle, aging, and environmental factors can have upon our body. They also eliminate free radicals. If you're interested in knowing the antioxidant power that essential oils possess, take a look at their ORAC (Oxygen Radial Absorption Capacity) amount indicated.For instance, the clove essential oil's ORAC value is 078 700 uTE/100g. This is quite high when as compared to carrots, which is 200 UTE/100g.

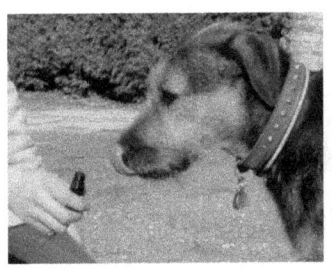

They ease digestion

Essential oils are known to help ease digestion. Peppermints, also are known as Mentha Piperita are great herbs well-known for their ability to soothe digestive issues. They also aid in improve your digestion.

It is easy and convenient to make use of.

Essential oils are very practical in the sense that they can be used any time. Have you ever thought that it is possible to wear essential oils all day? Yes, it's true and it is possible to do this no matter where you are, whether at work or at home. It is possible to carry them around in your pockets. They are essential in massage , too. They will improve your levels of concentration and meditation.

This can be used for animals as well.

It's remarkable that the usage of essential oils isn't only restricted to humans. Animals have been found to react well to essential oils as well. Some excellent examples include horses and dogs. While there are limitations for cats, essential oils can be utilized on cats.

Are they safe to use?

Essential oils can be used to help restore balance in your body without damaging it. This is because they don't contain chemicals. However, it is important to select essential oils that are therapeutic grade and not fragrance grade ones since these are made from toxic chemicals.

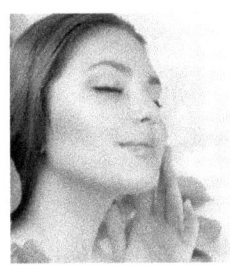

Multi-purpose

Essential oils have more than one use. For instance, the true lavender essential oil, also known as Lavandula angustifolia can be beneficial for minor burns and cuts because it's soft on the skin and has antimicrobial properties as well. It can also help promote relaxation and sleep when breathed in. So, you don't have to spend a lot of money on essential oils.

Essential oils refine your skin

Utilizing products for beauty that contain a lot of chemicals can erode the natural shine. But, if you turn to essential oils, you'll get your glow back. Essential oils can give your skin a fresh, healthy appearance.

Additionally they help minimize the appearance of aging signs and provide you with healthy hair.

Create deep spiritual awareness

Essential oils have been utilized in religious and spiritual ceremonies. They aid people in connecting with a higher entity higher than themselves. According to studies the essential oils contain molecules that activate Olfactory receptors. If you're looking to improve your spiritual experiences, then you can dilute essential oils, and then apply them on your wrists, feet and behind your ears. Or allow them to diffuse in a peaceful space in which you wish to experience your meditation.

Chapter 14: What to Take Care of Your Essential Oils

Essential oils are more than just their function. In reality the method by which they were made as well as how they are stored and stored has a significant impact on the effectiveness of their effects. be. If you want your essential oils to keep their optimal state, Here are some things to keep in mind.

Storage

Essential oils should be stored in a cool and dry location.

Certain substances are sensitive. Be cautious about where you put them.

* You can keep the oils in your refrigerator, or in other areas that aren't likely to occur.

For containers, it's recommended to store them in cobalt or amber blue bottles. Amber bottles are less expensive than blue ones.

Don't put the rubber dropper inside the bottle. Make sure you use an open cap to ensure that your oils remain secure and fresh.

Disposal

Essential oils can be extremely volatile. Do not dispose of them in flames.

* It is also recommended to flush all the oils in your drains, especially when there's a risk for the oil to come into contact with the water supply.

A few of the most suggested methods of disposing essential oils is to pour the oil into an inert object , and then sealing the two in the container of your choice.

Another option is to allow an essential oil's vapor to escape over baking soda.

If you have some essential oil there is the possibility to use it to use it for another use. You can make use of a tiny amount to help freshen your drain. Although pouring a lot of oil down the drain isn't recommended but a tiny portion of that oil isn't a bad idea also. It is possible to examine this amount against the ingredients that soap and skin care products contain which is flushed through the drain after you shower or wash your body. shower.

It is also possible to apply any remaining essential oils to dress your seasonal clothes. This will keep the bad smell from lingering until you're ready wear the clothing again. Cabinets and storage containers are also benefited by the oil. It's also possible to make use of this same product to scent your garbage bin. To enhance the scent from your washing, make a home-made fabric softener.

Reusing old essential oil bottles

There are numerous ways to recycle the bottles of essential oils you have discarded. If you're thinking of recycling it to make your new batch of essential oils it is important to ensure that there's nothing left of the previous contents. Here's how to thoroughly clean your bottles

Get the labels removed on the top of the bottle. Try to peel them off as many labels as you can.

Remove the bottles and their caps. Immerse everything in warm water for a few minutes.

To get rid of the sticky labels completely, add a few drops lemon oil into the water.

After the labels are thoroughly removed After soaking them, rinse them with another bowl of water using the aid of a household cleaner.

Cleanse the caps and bottles and let them dry in the air.

There are many exciting and innovative ways to recycle your bottles. It's not always about using them to make essential oils. For more ideas you can use, here's a brief list to consider:

Bottles that are old can serve as gift boxes. It is a great way to share essential oils or other homemade creations with your family and friends.

* You could use it to store your items for when you travel. It's not fun to take large bags and bags to hold your entire assortment of essential oils traveling across the country.

* These containers are also great for the storage of your homemade bath salts.

Chapter 15: The Power Of Smell

Did you realize that our perceptions of our fellows are largely dependent on our personal scent in addition to the appearance of our bodies or behaviour or communication abilities? It's not only a idea. Studies have repeatedly proven that each of us has our own distinctive scent (though often we don't even know it) that can cause us to appear more attractive or not to those in the vicinity. The way we smell communicates details about ourselves which is then taken into consideration by others. Contrary to contemporary advertising, our personal "basic" scent isn't altered by the use of scents, aftershaves and deodorants, or scented body washes. At maximum, we are able to disguise it for a short period of time.

The importance of smells is evident in a variety of industries, including wine-making, perfumery coffee roasting, food production, tobacco and cosmetics to name some of the most evident ones.The sense of smell is not just of the feeling of the odors but also of the experience and emotions that accompany the sensations. There is a strong connection between the smells, emotions and memories.Smell experiences are relayed to the brain's cortex and this is where recognition that is 'cognitive' takes place after the most profound areas of our brains are stimulated. Therefore when we are able to correctly identify a specific scent, such as"vanilla," the smell has already stimulated the limbic system, which triggers deeper emotional responses and memories that last for a long time. That is why many people suddenly and vividly recall distant memories when exposed to certain scents - the perfume worn by their mother, for example, can remind them of childhood.Certain aromas affect us psychologically; the smell of lemon is said to increase our perception of personal wellbeing.Supermarkets use the smell of freshly baked bread to make us feel hungry and buy more food, the smell of frankincense incense in a church can help us to feel more relaxed and in touch with our spiritual side.

Aroma is a word that refers to scent Therapy refers to treatment. Aromatherapy is a treatment that relies on the potential of smells. It comes from the practice of ancient times of using plant essences that are natural to boost health and wellbeing. Natural essences can be found in many components that comprise the plants, such as its leaves, flowers roots, wood seeds, fruits and bark in the form of

Essential oil(these are plant essential oils, also known as aroma-producing oils). Essential oils contain concentrations of the plants' healing properties and the same qualities that traditional Western medical practices employ in numerous medicines.

Aromatherapy is the practice of making use of these healing properties making use of the pure essential oils extracted from a variety of plants that are steam-distilled as well as cold-pressed out of flowers fruits, bark, and even roots.

The oils are extracted careful from certain parts of the plant such as the flower at specific times during the growth cycle.Potentially huge amounts of plant material are required to create small amounts of essential oils. Around 150 kg of lavender is needed for one Liter of essential lavender oil. This is why essential oils can be costly however, only small amounts of these essential oils are needed for beneficial effects.

Professional aromatherapists concentrate particular on the controlled application of essential oils for treating diseases and ailments, and to enhance physical and emotional well-being. There are three ways of working within your body. They are pharmacological which alters the chemical composition of the body, physiological, which impacts the body's ability to perform and function also, psychological. It influences moods and emotions. These three modes are constantly in contact. Aromatherapy is so effective because it influences the three modes:

Physiological effects:

The majority of essential oils possess antiseptic properties. They are able to fight off infections. They also help ease an variety of physical ailments that include burning, aches in the joints, pains, infections excessive blood pressure break down mucus, and open nasal passages, help digestion and increase blood circulation.

The effects of pharmacology:

They increase your immune system as well as the production of hormones such as insulin.

Psychological effects:

Aromatherapy can promote relaxation and reduce stress. Aromatherapy can also affect the nervous system of the central nerves, which can ease anxiety and depression, and making it less stressful by soothing, elevating, sedating or stimulating, and restoring mental and physical health.

Research is increasingly showing, the effects of smells all sorts of things, from emotions and dreams driving, stress and gambling, as well as pain concentration, memory, and love. Let's look at some scenarios in real life where aromatherapy has been proven efficient.

Stress and insomnia

According to a study by Maryland University, clinical trials have proven that the scent of lavender may help with anxiety, insomnia stress, after-operative pain." The research has evidence from science to suggest that lavender aromatherapy could decrease the activities of the nervous system, enhance the quality of sleep, improve relaxation and improve spirits in those who suffer from sleep disorders," according to the researchers. Vanilla, coffee, chamomile and roses all have similar calming effects. A Thailand study revealed that the aroma of roses has a positive effect on blood pressure and breathing.

Aromatherapy also has an enormous impact on our moods. A whiff of clary Sage is a good example. It can calm anxiety, and the aroma released by peeling an orange could make you feel more positive. Because your mind is a major influence on your health, and is an effective healing tool which can make aromatherapy even more thrilling.

Dreams

A pleasant scent before bed could lead to better dreams. Research has shown that emotions in later dreams was related to the scent. People with a pleasant scent (like for example rosewood, sandalwood) were significantly more likely to have positive dreams than those who did not have a smell, and those who had a bad smell (like sulfur) experienced the worst dreams.

Concentration

Spraying lavender scent during tea breaks in factories during tea breaks in Japan has been found to boost post-break productivity. People who smelled peppermint performed faster and were more focused than those with no scent, and children did better in tests when exposed to the scent of fresh strawberries.

Memory

Aromas can be powerful triggers of particular memories. They can be used in therapy to aid in the recovery of lost memories. Studies conducted at Toronto University shows that memories stimulated by the scents of clary sage or rosemary tend to be more clear as well as more intense and emotional.

Spending

The smell of a scent can have an impact on the products we purchase as well as how much we spend as well as on the way we wager on. One study was conducted in the Las Vegas casino, there was nearly 50% increase in wagers made when a pleasant scent applied to slot machines. Researchers from Chicago University found that 84 percent of customers were able to find identical shoes more appealing when they were placed in a space with an aroma that was pleasant as opposed to a room that was not scented. They also appreciated the shoes for PS10 more.

Nearly all essential oils provide numerous benefits, so keeping a half-a-dozen will assist you in treating a vast variety of common physical and emotional issues - and this is the appeal of aromatherapy.

For example,

Essential oil of Frankincense (commonly used to fight stress) gives the scent of a warm and relaxing that helps to ease asthmatic breathing.

Jasmine can help you improve your mood and ease depression and stress. Jasmine has also been utilized to treat aphrodisiacs.

Bergamot essential oil is sweet and fruity, with a citrus scent can relieve symptoms of depression. It can also aid in digestion, and aid in reducing tension in muscles.

There are hundreds of essential oils available Many of them will assist you to relax and deal with difficult situations in a more effective way. You might need to test to determine what oils are most beneficial for you. While lavender scents release positive feelings, a smudge of eucalyptus could boost your alertness.

Chapter 16: Purchase and Storing Essential oils

Since essential oils are utilized mostly for health and wellness and wellness, it is crucial to buy them from trusted vendors. Insufficient quality or adulterated oils are not going to give you the advantages you seek and can even cause harm. These tips will put you in good stead when aiding you in making the best choice.

Do not purchase items that say "fragrance oil,"" "perfume oil" or "nature similar oil" because they will not be pure essential oils.

Don't purchase from sellers who claim that their primary oils have the designation of "aromatic quality" or "therapeutic grade" since there isn't such thing.

* Only purchase essential oils from sellers who sell sizes of four oz. or less in dark

glass containers , not clear glass or plastic ones.

Purchase from vendors that offer adequate information on the product offered by them.

Beware of sellers that sell all types of essential oils for the same price.

Make sure to check the essential oils the botanical name, the location of extraction, as well as extraction process prior to buying.

• Be prepared with details about essential oils that are contained within the FDA guidelines for the essential oils as well as aromatherapy.

In terms of the proper the storage and preservation of essential oils, one must take into consideration that a lot oils are extremely fragile and are susceptible to degrade when exposed to sunlight, air or a high temperatures. Simple precautions can prevent that from happening.

Use the correct bottle Dark glass bottles are best to choose.

Make sure you use the right caps: Screw-on caps are the most effective to utilize.

A stable and secure environment to store your items: Avoid sunlight.

Keep them in a cool location They can be stored within the fridge (not on the counter in the freezer).

Avoid the source of heat. Keeping them near a fireplace, stove, or flame is a no-no since these oils are typically extremely flammable.

How do I use Essential Oils - Safety

Essential oils can be viewed as risky substances because they contain substances that have chemical components that are extremely concentrated. If treated in a responsible method, the risks associated with making use of essential oils are reduced. It is essential that you are aware of possible dangers and adhere to the basic guidelines when making use of essential oils. These tips will ensure your safety when making use of essential oils. If you're still uncertain of the best way to use the oil, it is recommended to speak with a doctor or an aromatherapist.

Due to their potent nature, it is necessary to be careful when making use of essential oils. Here are the security precautions you should follow when making use of essential oils:

If you are using it for bathing: It is recommended to first dilute essential oils using emulsifiers, such as milk or sesame oils to assist in dispersing them and stop the development of derma toxins due to the oils floating in hot water that comes into close contact with skin. In addition the care must be taken to use only essential oils suitable for bathing, such as rose oil, lavender oil clary sage oil sandalwood oil, geranium oil, cedar oil pine oil and others. Five to 10 drops of essential oils mixed with half to a complete cup of emulsifier will be enough to fill a bath.

If used to inhale: Care should be taken not to inhale for long periods of period of time as it could cause a variety of issues such as headaches, dizziness nausea, lethargy , and even vertigo.The dose should not exceed 10 drops of essential oil when inhaled with diffusers or heating water. If you are using a steam facial the dosage should be 5 to 1 drop in a water pot.

If used to massage because of their abundant nature essential oils should be properly diluted to make suitable for massages. The recommended dose for children who are less than 12 years old will be six drops in ounce. and for adults 15 drops per oz.

Essential oils shouldn't be applied undiluted to the skin There are situations where people who have experience using essential oils do make exceptions. But, there are a lot of risks to applying essential oils that are not diluted to the skin. It is not recommended to do it without a thorough understanding of the hazards because essential oils are extremely concentrated, and every component of the oil reacts in a different way to the skin. There are instances where someone could apply an essential oil without diluting or undiluted, can result in the possibility of a bug bite, burn or irritation. If you choose to apply an essential oil for this purpose it is crucial to be aware that you should not use essential oils on a child without mixing the oil.

Certain oils could lead allergies in a few people , or may cause skin sensitivity when you apply the application of a new oil at first, it's essential to conduct a patch test using a small portion of the skin before applying the entire area. The process of sensitization happens when you are vulnerable to reactions from an essential oil you have never previously experienced a reaction to. If you notice that you're suddenly experiencing a reaction to an essential oil and stop using it, you should discontinue it.

What to do for an To Perform a Skin Patch Test: Performing a skin patch test is simple and is essential to determine if an essential oils will trigger the skin's reaction. Be aware that no matter how much you do not react to a specific essential oil does not mean that others might not react. Remember that if you're sensitive to a certain plant, you're more than likely to be allergic to the essential oil of that plant.

* Apply one to two drops of essential oil that has been diluted in the elbow area of your hand. (Diluted is when the essential oil is blended with carrier oil)

* Use a bandage, or gauze to the area to make sure that the area is not submerged throughout the testing.

If you experience any reaction or irritation immediately take off the bandage and clean the area thoroughly with mild soap and water.

* If there isn't any irritation after 24 hours, the dilute essential oil can be used to apply it to your skin.

Some essential oils are toxic Essential oils that are phototoxic may cause irritation, inflammation burning, redness and blisters when exposed to UVA radiation. The citrus oils in a particular group can be considered toxic. There are however some exceptions to the rule. Here is an overview of the essential citrus oils that aren't phototoxic.

Lemon, steam distilled;

Lime, steam distilled;

Mandarin;

Sweet Orange

Tangerine and

Furocoumarin/bergapten free Bergamot

There are times when you Should Not Use Essential Oils There are essential oils to be avoided if pregnant, suffer from epilepsy, asthma or other medical conditions. Make sure you consult with your doctor or a certified professional before making use of any essential oil in case you suffer from any health concerns or health worries regarding using essential oils.

A little is more Essential oils are highly concentrated. If a recipe requires between one and two drops of essential oil, it is all you're going to need to complete the task completed. Always ensure that you use the carrier oil when you're applying essential oils on your skin.

Certain essential oils are not appropriate for use in aromatherapy Certain oils that aren't designed to be used in aromatherapy. They are wintergreen, rue onion bitter almond, wormwood and bitter almond. Use only essential oils that have been recommended to be used in aromatherapy. If you're not sure it is best to consult a certified practitioner before using.

Essential oils should not be Consumed in the body: due to the high amount of essential oil, these shouldn't be consumed without having a clear knowledge of the risks and usage that come with every oil.

Essential oils can ignite: Protect your essential oils from hazards that could ignite.

Some quick pointers on using Essential Oils

Essential oils are typically extremely concentrated. This is why they are somewhat risky to apply them randomly. It is important to make sure that you're able manage your own body and the oils that you choose to use when you've made the decision to use them on your body. There are certain rules you must adhere to. They are explicitly mentioned in this portion in the book.

It is always recommended to make use of a drop-sized orifice. You must ensure that you're using the right amount of oil, based on the amount that is recommended by your physician or the expert you've been talking to. When you have children in your home, it is important to make sure that there is an opening which only reduces the amount of drop. That way, your child or you do not utilize more than is needed. If you discover that the child or you has taken more than what is required then you must consult a doctor right away. Butbefore you leave to the doctor, drink a glass of milk.

Before you use the oil to your children, consult a physician to confirm the use of the oil on your children. It is always advisable to be aware of any potential repercussions.

Before beginning to use essential oils, you'll have to make sure that they don't harm your skin. It is essential to ensure the skin protected when using this essential oil. It is recommended to try the oil on the skin with a small patch. Follow the steps previously mentioned. If you notice that the oil has damaged your skin even a tiny bit be sure to remove the oil immediately.

It is always best to utilize oils as blends since using the oils in isolation may not produce an intended effect.The methods in the cookbook make use of mixtures of several oils. It is recommended to try these blends as well. Apply a tiny amount of oil to your skin, and then wait some time. If you observe that there isn't any negative reaction towards the product, you may keep using it.

Essential oils can affect any object , and could also harm your skin. If you notice that you've applied essential oils and then touched to your lenses with your fingers, you could be causing permanent damage to them. Additionally, you could harm your eyes through the process. Get rid of the lenses as soon as possible then apply 2 drops of oil from a vegetable on your eyes.

You must be extremely cautious about your ears. Beware of applying essential oils near your ears.

Essential oils produce different effects when they are in the sun as well as in darkness. If you are one who is frequently on the move then it would be beneficial to know the effects of various oil types on the body, especially when you're out in the sunlight.

Don't apply essential oils to your skin if there is makeup applied over it. The oil will get absorbed into your skin by the makeup. It is crucial to keep in mind that essential oils enter the bloodstream quickly.

Essential oils should not be used on a bruised burnt, scarred, or burned skin due to the reasons listed in the previous paragraphs. Additionally, it can cause the wound to become more septic, leading to an additional kind of problem.

Chapter 17: Eucalyptus Oil

To Lose Weight: Eucalyptus oil comes from the dried leaves of the eucalyptus plant which is a native evergreen from Australia.Eucalyptus was used for centuries to treat against colds, fevers and body pains . Today it's both an established defender of inflammation and an anti-infection agent.When it concerns weight loss, eucalyptus oil offers an essential boost in any diet program to reduce inflammation in the system. When the inflammation-related conditions of your body are cooled and your metabolism improves, you are and can work at full efficiency, leading to weight reduction. Eucalyptus oil is an excellent anti-fungal remedy, and if you suspect you have a fungal infection in your system, such as candida may be the reason for your swelling, bloating as well as weight loss, taking a breath of this essential oil will reduce the amount of fungal burden in your body swiftly and effortlessly.

Candida is also known for its ability to cause weight gain through the increase in your desire for carbohydrates and sugary foods, but the ability of eucalyptus oil to regulate the body's hunger signals can aid you in fighting to this delightful hunger.For rapid hunger control, spray or soak two cotton balls with eucalyptus oils and store them in the form of a Ziploc bag. If you notice that hunger signals are beginning to set in, grab a cotton ball and breathe in the aroma. The cravings will decrease rapidly and you can take better food choices instead of being restricted by candida.

For Pain Relief:Eucalyptus oil is a demonstrated analgesic, pain relieving properties.Studies have proven that placing dilute eucalyptus oil onto those areas where pain is felt can result in a significant reduction of strains and aches. It's also possible to use the oil to aid in pain prevention by massaging the oil in your muscles prior to a workout. The natural warmth that comes from the oil can help your muscles warm up and protect them from straining or pulling, regardless of how much you work out.

for stress relief and mental Rejuvenation: If you're stressed or want to improve your brain's abilities to complete a task or test, eucalyptus oil can provide the perfect anxiety-reducing and rejuvenating effect.It can reduce tension, stress and tired mind by releasing an uplifting and refreshing scent. By inhaling steam from eucalyptus, you will increase the flow of blood to your brain, allowing you concentrate more fast and precisely. When you next need to focus on a school or work-related task, you can make use of a nebulizer that produces steam from eucalyptus and take numerous deep breaths within an interval from 12 to 12 inches.

To help in reducing the smell and ease of breathing If you suffer from seasonal allergies or suffer from an unending congestion of your nose, eucalyptus oil could be your ideal companion. Its strong scent can clear obstructions in the nasal or moth, as well as in the chest area and allows you to breathe better. When it opens your nasal passages, it can also clear any mucus that is backed up and is therefore an essential option to treat colds, flus, and other respiratory diseases such as bronchitis. If you're struggling to breathe, try Eucalyptus oil instead prescription medication. You will be amazed at the immediate results you will see!

Aromatherapy:

While nebulizing and diffusion are both excellent options for eucalyptus oils, the most effective and healing technique to use it is to use it in a warm body bath. Take a bath in warm water with 7 to 8 drops the oil of eucalyptus to be mixed in the bath by placing the oil into the water flowing. After the oil has been absorbed, relax at a warm temperature for about 30 minutes. While you soak, you should focus on taking in the strong eucalyptus aroma into your lungs.

If you're dealing with an area that is particularly sore or strain you can gently massage the eucalyptus oil-scented bath water onto the skin that covers the problematic region. Since eucalyptus oil is known to have an effect of cooling it is recommended that this bath be taken in cooler conditions. In colder seasons be sure to avoid entering an air-conditioned room right after taking an bath with eucalyptus oil since the cooling effect could be multiplied, resulting in the body temperature dropping drastically.

In order to eliminate Mites as well as Insects:

If you're dealing with an bed bug or insect infestation however you do not want to employ harsh chemicals at home, consider nebulizing the essential oils of eucalyptus in the area. You could also spray carpet or furniture by using a concentrated solution of eucalyptus oil as well as water. Add between 8 and 10 drops of oil from eucalyptus per 1 cup of water. Stir thoroughly and then spray the affected area with the mixture. The bugs, ticks and mites that you're dealing with will either go away or attempt to leave the area immediately.You could also utilize the oil of eucalyptus as a pest repellent in your garden. In order to get rid of bugs, mites and white flies, and other pests make a mixture of 1 drop of eucalyptus oil and 1/3 cup water. Put the mixture in the spray bottle and shake. Spray this mixture into the soil and mulch around the plants that are being attacked pests in the garden or directly on the plants and you will notice a decrease in aphids, bugs and other garden dangers.

Beware of the following: Eucalyptus oil is one of the oldest and extensively used essential oils of all, and is among the safest oils, too. However, there are few precautions you should be aware of when making use of it. I recommend adults use eucalyptus oil either topically or in breath form. It is best to use it orally when you are in medical care. Eucalyptus oil is extremely concentrated and therefore it could be too powerful for your system and could even cause harm when taken in large enough dosages.

Do not let your children consume eucalyptus oil, and keep it away from their reach. Eucalyptus oil can be safe for use on the skin, however it shouldn't be used on children because their skin is more sensitive than the adult skin. Small animals can also get sick when they consume the oil. Therefore, avoid rooms and areas which are treated with a eucalyptus solution. Women who are pregnant or nursing shouldn't use eucalyptus oil. If you apply the oil on your garden plants ensure that pets don't consume any treated mulch, soil or leaves.

Chapter 18: The Essential Oils and Their Beneficial Effects

Essential oils offer many advantages. They are often used to fragrance, incense, or as a mood boosters. Essential oils have a variety of advantages and properties that can be utilized for various purposes.

They are typically blended together, leading to a wide variety of combinations with a variety of applications. They are often paired by their advantages or smell. Be aware that these are extremely potent oils and could cause irritation in people with sensitive skin or are sensitive to scents. Conduct a patch test on your skin prior to using any essential oil to avoid any problems.

Allspice

The oil is made from Pimenta dioica belonging to the Myrtaceae family. It is commonly referred to as Jamica Pepper, Pimenta or Pimento Oil. The tree is an evergreen plant that is located throughout South America and West Indies.

It is warm and cosy with a sweet, spicy smell. It is a taste of clove paired with juniper berries, cinnamon and pepper. It helps to alleviate pain, create numbness and calm the body, increase bodily functions and add some color to your skin. It's an analgesic antiseptic stimulant, anesthetic and tonic, relaxant rubefacient and carminative.

It is well paired with ginger, geranium lavender, orange, patchouli clove, cassia, cinnamon, ylang ylang, and.

Angelica

Angelica has a pleasant scent with a hint of spice. It is derived from Angelica archangelica, a plant that is found to Eastern Europe. It blooms typically on May 8th, that coincides with St. Michael's Day, an archangel. This is why it is planted most often in monasteries and is known as Angel Grass, giving it its name Angelica.

It helps to boost the lymphatic system, and cleanses the body. It also serves as a powerful treatment for respiratory conditions as well as issues with stomach issues, such as dyspepsia flatulence, indigestion, and nausea. It can be useful for treating skin irritations, psoriasis dull skin, arthritis, gout as well as bronchitis, rheumatism as well as cough, water retention anemia, anorexia headache, fatigue, stress and tension.

Although it blends well with the essential oils in a aromatic way, it is most effective when blended with mandarin, patchouli grapefruit, lavender, lemon Geranium, chamomile, and basil. It is commonly utilized in vaporizers and burners massage oil, the bath, and is also mixed with lotions and creams.

Aniseed

The oil is spicy and warm. It is extracted from the fruit as well as seeds from Pimpinella anisum, which is an herb that was discovered in the Middle East. It is also referred to as sweet cumin, but it is not to be mistaken for star anise however they both have similar liqourice-like scents.

The oil can be beneficial for the respiratory tract, digestive system and circulation system. It eases hangover catarrh and flatulence menstrual cramps and colic, whooping cough muscle pains, bronchitis, and rheumatism.

Be cautious when using this oil. In large doses, it can result in cerebral congestion. Women who are pregnant should not use the oil.

It's a good match It is well paired with Cedarwood Caraway, cardamom coriander, dill mandarin and fennel, as well as petitgrain and rosewood.

Basil

It is a mild yellowish-greenish hue and is characterized by a sweet, spicy and green scent. It is frequently employed in aromatherapy to calm your mind, relax the nerves, relieve congestion in the sinuses, reduce the fever, and help treat issues with menstrual flow.

It's used to treat asthma and bronchitis and nausea, constipation, vomiting and hiccups. It typically refreshes the skin and is also used for acne and bites from insects.

It is well paired with black pepper as well as bergamot, Cedarwood and ginger. It is also a great blend with fennel Geranium, grapefruit marjoram, lavender, lemon verbena and neroli.

Benzoin

It is a resinous oil that comes by the Styrax Benzoin plant from Sumatra, Java and Thailand. It's also known as gum benzoin Benjamin Luban Jawi, the styrax benzoin.

It's golden brown hue and a warm, sweet vanilla-like scent. It's a relaxing oil that lifts spirits and calms the mind. It provides comfort to those who feel lonely and sad. It also helps to heal cracked skin and increases its elasticity. It also helps heal wounds, sores and itching. It can also be used to treat eczema, acne and psoriasis. It also helps heal scars and digestive issues, circulation issues and respiratory tract disorders.

It is well-suited to the bergamot scent, coriander, frankincense as well as juniper, lavender Myrrh, lemon petitgrain as well as sandalwood, orange and rose.

Bergamot

The fresh, citrus-yet-fresh sweet, spicy-floral, fruity-sour oil is made from Citrus aurantium Varieties. bergamia, which is also known as the bergamot orange. It gives you a calm and happy sensation, which makes it a top choice for aromatherapists.

It helps relieve tension, stress and depression. It also helps with anorexia, depression anxiety and hysteria. It can also help treat the symptoms of eczema and psoriasis as well skin acne, chicken pox as well as cold sores and wounds.

It's a great blend with the black pepper, cypress, clary sage and frankincense. jasmine, geranium and nutmeg mango, orange, rosemary, sandalwood, ylang-ylang and vetiver.

Black Pepper

This spicy, sharp-tasting oil is made from Piper nigerum , a member of the Piperaceae family. It soothes the body as well as the mind and increases circulation. It also helps improve digestion and also stimulates the colon and kidneys. It also boosts appetite and eases sore muscles, pain , and fever.

It is well-mixed with clove, bergamot coriander, clary sage the fennel, frankincense Geranium, grapefruit lemon and lime, lavender mandarin, juniper and ylang-ylang.

Cajuput

It comes from Melaleuca cajuputi. This is an evergreen tree that is often referred to as weeping trees, wood with white, or weeping paperback. It helps balance the mind, helps clear thoughts and helps to reduce an euphoria. It has a pleasant, penetrating smell that is often employed in cosmetics and perfumes.

It helps cool the body, promoting perspiration and assists in relieving bronchitis, laryngitis, colds and coughs. It also assists in curing the symptoms of sinusitis, sore throat, and asthma. It also aids in digestion, arthritis muscular pains, and arthritis. Its antiseptic properties aid in battling skin infections like acne and psoriasis. It also helps to relieve bites caused by lice and other insects and stops them from coming back too.

It is a great blend with bergamot angelica Geranium, cloves Thyme, lavender and angelica.

Roman Camomile or Chamomile

It is taken from Anthemis nobelis, which is part of the species family Asteraceae. It is sometimes referred to as garden-chamomile sweet chamomile, English chamomile.

The oil is a bit watery, with the color of clear blue and has a scent that resembles sweet apple. It is a wonderful calming effect, which makes it a great choice for kids who are struggling with teeth, angry and anxious. It also helps with PMS as well as gall bladder issues and abdominal pain, allergies asthma, throat infections and the hay fever. It can also help relieve urinary stones and all forms of inflammation.

It's a good match with clary sage, bergamot lavender, geranium tree, jasmine grapefruit, ylang ylang and lemon.

Camphor

The oil is extracted by the Camphor tree. Be careful when choosing the camphor essential oil. Make sure to use only white camphor with a clean smell and clear aroma. Don't use the yellow version since it is a source of safrole which can cause cancer and is harmful.

The oil helps to balance your mood. It also calms nerves and boosts your mood. It eases discomfort, cold cough, bronchitis and other cold symptoms. It also repels insects like moths and Flies. It also aids in relieving muscular injuries, sprains, arthritis and arthritis.

It is a great blend with lavender, cajuput basil, chamomile and Melissa.

Cedarwood

The balsamic oil comes from Juniperus virginiana Also called Bedford Cedarwood Lebanon cedar. It's viscous, with a an orange-yellow to pale yellow color, and a woody pencil-like scent with the scent of sandalwood.

It is particularly beneficial for skin because of its sedative effects. It is able to treat the appearance of acne and oily skin, and itching. It can also be effective in treating chest infections, dandruff and urinary tract infections. It also relaxes and soothes the mind, assisting when it comes to conditions that cause anxiety and nervous tension.

It is well-suited to benzoin, cypress, bergamot and jasmine. It is also a good blend with cinnamon as well as juniper, frankincense lavender as well as lemon, neroli rosemary , and rose.

Cinnamon

It comes from Cinnamomum Zeylanicum, which is often referred to as real cinnamon Ceylon and Seychelles. It is a smoky and spicy scent that aids in calming anxiety, relieve feelings of fatigue, and combats weakness.

In the ancient times of Egypt It was used to massage the feet as a treatment for bile excess and also as a temple incense. It can also be used as a an sedative for babies and as a main ingredient in love potion and mulled wine.

It is best to avoid this oil during pregnancy because of its emmenagogue effect. Only the essential oil of the leaves can be used to treat aromatherapy. The cinnamon oil extracted from bark may cause irritation, is a source of dermal toxins, and also sensitizer.

It's used to clear warts, soothing the respiratory tract as well as the nervous system. It reduces the symptoms of colds and flu.

It is well paired with coriander, cloves, benzoin ginger, cardamom, cloves, frankincense rosemary, lavender and Thyme.

Citronella

The oil is made from a perennial tough grass that is indigenous in Java as well as

Sri Lanka. It is an acknowledged repellent to insects and is widely used for clearing the mind, cleansing the sickroom, softening skin, fights the oily skin and soothes sweaty feet.

It has a citrusy lemony scent with an underlying sweetness. It is commonly used in candles, lotions, perfumes deodorants and soaps. It's also beneficial for treating colds, infections and influenza.

It is well paired with bergamot and geranium lemon, orange pine, and lavender.

Clary Sage

The extracts oil from flowers and leaves of the biennial plant. It's sometimes referred to as clary wort as well as muscatel sage, and see bright. Its scent is sweet and nutty with a herbal undertone.

It relaxes your nervous system which makes it beneficial in treatment of tension, depression, insomnia , and anxiety. It also serves to help relax babies. It eases discomfort in the muscles, kidney disorders and digestive issues. It also helps reduce skin inflammation such as boils, ulcers and acne. It regulates the production of sebum on the skin, which eliminates oil and cleanses the skin's complexion.

It's a great blend with juniper, lavender sandalwood, pine, geranium jasmine, frankincense, jasmine, along with citrus oils.

Dill

The oils is obtained from seeds or from the whole plant. This is an annual weed that originates to South West Asia. It has a pale yellow color as well as an earthy, natural-smelling smell.

It eases the feeling of feeling overwhelmed and helps calm the mind. It's beneficial for digestive issues as well as for Hiccups. It also assists in reducing excessive sweating caused by anxiety and tension. Breastfeeding mothers will profit from this oil since it aids in increasing the amount of breast milk produced.

It is well paired with citrus fruits, as well as caraway and nutmeg and the bergamot.

Eucalyptus

The oil comes out of the Australian blue gum tree which is also called Tasmanian blue gum. It is distinctive and has a fresh, clean scent that can help focus the mind and aids in greater concentration and focus.

It can be very beneficial in treating fever, migraines headaches, respiratory problems as well as muscle and skin problems such as skin lesions as well as wounds, congested skin and ulcers.

It is well-suited to blending with benzoin, thyme, pine, lemongrass and lavender.

Fennel

The oils is extracted by seeds from the perennial plant called Sweet Fennel,

Roman Fennel or Fenkle. Egyptians and Romans utilize fennel for strengthening their eyesight, and as a treatment for snakebite and get rid of the fleas that plague dogs. The belief is that it helps to keep from evil spirits, boost endurance and strength and increase endurance.

It has a strong, herbal scent that is spicy with a hint that is similar to aniseed. When consumed in large quantities it could cause negative narcotic impact and should be avoided when there is epilepsy or pregnancy.

This essential oil is employed to lose weight since it creates a feeling of fullness, and its diuretic properties help the body to eliminate the toxins. Aromatherapy is used to boost the courage and strength to take on life's challenges. It is also a source of estrogen that can aid in reducing wrinkles and clearing the skin, reduce oily skin and speed up the healing process of bruises. It aids in digestion problems and the occurrence of hiccups. It also improves the tone of the liver and spleen.

It is well paired together with sandalwood rose and lavender.

Frankincense

The oil is made by removing the resin from Boswellia carteri plant. It is also known as Olibanum. This has an appealing woody scent that is slightly spicy and camphorous.

The ancient times saw frankincense was utilized by Egyptians for face masks and as an offer to their Gods. Hebrews considered this oil to be highly valuable and offered it as a present to the newborn Jesus. Also, it was utilized to cast away evil spirits and purify the sick.

In aromatherapy, it's utilized to relax the mind and bring about peace within, making it a favourite among people who meditate and practicing yoga. It helps to calm obsessive thoughts and anxiety. It is also utilized in labor due to its relaxing effect. It also aids in easing pain and inflammation in urine flow. It also aids in improving the appearance of the skin, and also helps heal cuts, carbuncles and scars and inflammation of the skin.

It's a great blend with benzoin, bergamot as well as pine, lemon Myrrh, orange, and sandalwood.

Geranium

The oils is extracted by stalks and leaves of the plant.This plants has around 700 varieties. Only few of them yield a substantial quantity of oil. In the past, Geranium was planted around homes to keep spirits at bay.

Aromatherapy is a form of therapy. Geranium is among essential oils frequently employed. It helps to clear the mind and regulates hormones and emotional balance. Additionally, it stimulates lymphatic systems as well as the adrenal cortex.It helps keep the skin smooth and elastic while also managing sebum production to avoid acne.It is also helpful to heal cuts, wounds or cuts, eczema and dermatitis. It also helps to repel mosquitoes, lice and ringworms. It can also be used to combat breast insufflation, poor circulation and PMS.

It's a good match with basil, angelica carrot seeds, bergamot citrus, cedarwood, jasmine, sage, grapefruit lime, lavender rosemary, orange and neroli.

Grapefruit

The essential oil is extracted from the fresh peels of fruit that are then cold compressed. The grapefruit tree originates from Asia and is currently grown across Israel, Brazil and the USA.

It has a significant impact on the body, which makes it useful in counteracting tension, depression, fatigue and stiffness. It also acts as diuretic, which helps the body eliminate the toxins and eliminate cellulite. It also aids in treating acne and oily skin, and helps to promote hair growth.

It's a good match with geranium, bergamot lavender, frankincense along with Palma Rosa.

Jasmine

The essential oil comes through the flowering of the evergreen plant which was first discovered within Northern India and China. For the best results, flowers should be picked in the night because the scent is most intense at this time.

It calms nerves and is a great treatment for depression. The floral, sweet exotic scent of this oil gives an euphoric feeling, confidence and optimism. It also helps to restore the energy lost. It's also helpful in managing post-natal depression, and aids in the production of milk. It can also help ease muscular pains and respiratory problems. It improves the skin's elasticity, which reduces stretching marks, scars and stretch marks.

It's a great blend with citrus oil, bergamot sandalwood and rose.

Lavender

It comes from the flowers of the evergreen plant known by the name of English lavender, commonly known as and garden lavender. The fresh, pleasant scent of Lavender soothes the mind and relaxes body, making it ideal for relieving anxiety and stress, as well as fighting against crises.

Its antiseptic properties aid in easing colds, flu, fever asthma, bronchitis whooping cough, throat infection and halitosis. It also aids in relieving joint and muscle pains. It can help with all kinds of skin issues. It is also a great insect repellent.

It's a great blend with cedarwood, clary Sage, pine, geranium, and all citrus oils, and the spice nutmeg.

Lemon

The essential oil comes from the fresh peels of fruit through the cold process. The fresh, crisp citrus scent of lemon improves concentration and helps improve decision-making. In Japan banks make use of the essential oils of lemon in their diffusers to prevent errors that are caused by employees. It's also a sought-after flavoring ingredient in food as well as a scent for perfumes.

The Middle Ages, an ounce of lemon was given by members of the Royal Navy each day to combat vitamin deficiencies, including Scurvy. It's beneficial for nosebleeds because it decreases blood pressure. It also aids in lowering fever as well as treat bronchitis, flu as well as throat infections.It helps with headaches, migraines and migraines as well as herpes, and insect bites. Its antibacterial and antiseptic properties aid in clearing the skin and rid it of acne. It also eliminates grease from hair and the skin.

It is well paired with elemi, benzoin, Fennel, eucalyptus and juniper. It also blends well with lavender, sandalwood, rose and neroli.

Marjoram

The extract is derived from flowers and leaves of the perennial bushy herb that is also called knotted marjoram. In the past, in Greece it was presented to newlyweds as a symbol to bring good luck. It was also extensively utilized by the Greeks for their perfume and medicine.

The spicy, yet warm scent of this oil soothes the mind and calms hyperactive people. It relieves stress and anxiety. It also relaxes muscles, making it beneficial for spasms, muscle pains strains, strains, and sprains. It also relaxes the digestive system, and helps relieve the symptoms that come with it. It can also help with headaches, migraines, insomnia and migraines. Note that marjoram is able to decrease sexual cravings.

It is well paired with cedarwood, chamomile the eucalyptus, cypress, bergamot tea tree and lavender.

Neroli

The oil is derived from the flowers of the bitter-orange plant, which is also known as orange blossom, flower, or neroli bigarade. Its refreshing, floral smell is a soothing affect on the mind as well as the body. It eases heart palpitations, reduces shock, depression and anxiety.

It aids in treating spasms, diarrhea, and colitis. It's very beneficial for skin health as it helps regenerate and rejuvenate skin cells. It reduces scarring, assists reduce stretch marks, treats damaged capillaries and helps to maintain the smoother appearance of skin.

It is well paired with geranium and lavender jasmine, benzoin sandalwood, rosemary, along with all the citrus oils.

Rosemary

It is extracted from the flowers of the evergreen shrub by steam distillation. In the Middle Ages, rosemary was used to prevent negative spirits. Its fresh, clear herbal scent promotes mental clarity and increases memory and stimulates your brain.

It also aids in treating jaundice as well as relieve joint and muscle discomforts. It also assists in reducing the retention of water and assists in the loss of weight and elimination of cellulite. It is widely employed for hair growth as well as treatment of the scalp and hair as it increases blood flow for the scalp and helps in thereby stimulating growth and improving health.

It's a great blend with cedarwood, citronella lemongrass, lavender and peppermint.

Sandalwood

It is taken from the woody core of the tree. It is a scented woody scent with an exotic, scent that soothes the mind and has the effect of harmonization. It also helps reduce anxiety and confusion, fears anxiety, stress, and chronic illness.

It can also be helpful for problems with the chest, bladder infections, as well as frigidity and impotence. It's also excellent for skin care because it helps to tone the skin, eases itching and inflammation, reduces skin scarring and fights eczema.

It is well-mixed with myrrh and vetiver, rose, ylang ylang, Geranium, bergamot, black pepper, and lavender.

Chapter 19: Nutmeg Essential Oil

Nutmeg is the fruit from a plant indigenous to the hot tropical regions. The fruit is utilized as a spice to flavor food items. The components of nutmeg are potent detoxifiers, and have been proven to provide long-term relief from respiratory ailments as well as digestive issues.

How to use the essential nutmeg oil:

The essential oil of Nutmeg can be consumed by mixing with honey or water. To treat infections on the outside, you must put the oil onto the skin. You can also diffuse it to experience the amazing scent from the essential oil.

Ingredients needed to make essential nutmeg oil:

*Groundnutmeg

*Olive oil

*Glass Jar with lid

*Aluminium foil

Double boiler

*Cheesecloth

How do you make essential nutmeg oil:

Make a single layer of cheesecloth to protect the ground nutmeg, and then tie the string around it to create a pouch. The pouch should be kept in the jar, and then add olive oil to it. Cover the lid with aluminum foil around the lid. This foil can prevent the escape of steam as well as oil during heating.

Then, place the jar into the double boiler. Add the sufficient water into the boiler. Now, heat it up on the stove. Set the boiler to boil for one hour and then store the jar unattended for about a week. The longer you keep it in this manner and the more amount of oil.

After you're done then pour the oil out by straining it through many layers of cheesecloth. Then put the oil into an opaque bottle. keep it in a cool, dry location.

Parsley Essential Oil

Parsley is an herb that smells delicious and is indigenous in the Mediterranean region. The components in parsley possess a powerful antiseptic properties. Essential oil of parsley is among the most well-known diuretic ingredients that aid in a greater amount of the amount of urine, which aids in eliminating the wastes from the your body.

How to make use of Parsley Essential Oil:

Parsley essential oil is consumed by mixing it with honey or water. It has a wonderful aroma. essential oil is able to be inhaled using diffusers.

Ingredients for making parsley essential oil:

Fresh parsley leaves

*Rice bran oil

*Cheesecloth

*Glass jar

How to make essential parsley oil:

To create this essential oil, you will need to make use of freshly cut parsley leaves. The leaves should be crushed using the aid of a pestle and mortar so that the leaves begin with the release of oil.

Fill the jar in glass with oil from rice bran, and place the chopped parsley into the jar. Then seal the jar and place it in a spot in which there is ample sunlight and warmth. It should be left unattended for at the very least for one week.

Pour the oil into the dark bottle, after straining it through many layer of cheesecloth. The oil must be kept in a dry and cool location.

Patchouli Essential Oil

Patchouli can be described as an evergreen tree belonging to the Labiatae family. It is closely with lavender, mint and sage. The scent from this essential oil can be described as wonderful that is why it has a powerful affect on mood. The ingredients in this plant and their flowers can kill the fungus, and are widely employed as anti-fungal medicines. In addition, taking this oil can provide relief from flu and cold.

How do you use essential oil of patchouli:

Patchouli essential oil directly to external fungal diseases. To treat flu and cold ailments, the oil is to be taken in conjunction with honey or water.

Ingredients to make essential oils of patchouli:

*Fresh patchouli leaves

*Fresh patchouli flower.

*Rice bran oil

*Cheesecloth

*Glass jar

How to make essential patchouli oil:

In order to make this essential oil, you will need to only use fresh patchesouli leaves and flowers. They should be crushed using the aid of a mortar and pestle, until they begin in releasing oil.

Fill the glass the jar with the rice bran oils. keep the crushed leaves of patchouli and the flowers inside. Close the jar and place it in a spot that it has plenty of sunshine and warmth. It must be left unattended for at minimum one week.

Then, pour the oil into an opaque bottle after straining it through multiple sheets of cheesecloth. The oil must be kept in a dry and cool area.

Pine Essential Oil

Pine is a popular coniferous plant with an earthy fragrance. The strong and dry scent of the pine essential oil differs from the oil made from pine nuts. The essential oils ingredients comprised of pine leaves can be helpful in relieving stiffness in muscles. It also has diuretic properties well. If taken regularly, it aids to increase urination levels and eliminates toxins from your body. The scent is certain to improve your mood.

How to make use of Essential oil of Pine:

The essential oil of pine can be consumed in conjunction with honey or water. Massage this oil into stiff and strained muscles. Inhaling the oil through a diffuser can provide wonderful scent benefits.

Ingredients needed to make essential oils from pine:

Fresh pine leaves and the twigs

*Rice bran oil

*Cheesecloth

*Glass jar

How do you make essential oil of pine:

To extract this essential oil , you have to make use of only freshly cut pine leaves as well as twigs. They should be crushed using a pestle and mortar until they begin in releasing oil.

Fill the jar in glass with oil from rice bran, and keep the wood twigs and pine leaves within the jar. Then seal the jar and place it in a location in which there is ample sunlight and warmth. It must remain in a quiet place for at the very least for one week.

Then, pour the oil into the dark bottle, after straining it through multiple sheets of cheesecloth. The oil must be kept in a cool , dry area.

Rosewood Essential Oil

Rosewood is an evergreen plant belonging to the laurel family. Essential oils are made using wood shavings. They possess a wonderful scent that is spicy and woody which aids in enhancing mood. The components of the essential oil rosewood have anti-fungal properties, which makes them useful in healing wounds. They will also give us relief from discomfort.

How to make use of essential oils of rosewood:

Rosewood essential oil can be inhaled using diffuser. To reap the benefits of anti-fungal you can apply a some drops of the oil on wounds and cuts.

Ingredients to make essential rosewood oil:

*Scrapings of rosewood

*Olive oil

*Glass jar

How do you make essential rosewood oil:

The glass jar will be filled with rosewood shavings to ensure that there's not much empty space.

Pour the olive oil until the rosewood shavings have been completely submerged in the oil.

The bottle should be stored in a warm area and ensure that it is warm during the entire day. This process should be followed for at minimum 3 weeks, and remember that you shake your bottle frequently.

After three weeks Pour the oil into a dark, clean bottle by straining it through several layers of cheesecloth. Keep it in a cool, dry area.

Conclusion

With all you've learned from this article the following step will be to apply this information into practice, and then to build your knowledge of essential oils more. Keep on your watch for more in-depth guides to aromatherapy and other natural solutions, geared towards people who have more experience.

Spend a few months now to begin building your collection of essential oils, gain knowledge and gain an understanding of the effects of each oil on your. When you are comfortable using the essential oils you are familiar with then you can begin to explore and use the lesser-known yet equally potent essential oils available there.

While essential oils are often considered to be an alternative to hazardous and poisonous prescriptions, their safety remains a concern. The potent oils are highly concentrated and could result in serious harm to your health when not utilized properly and in a responsible manner. To demonstrate how intense these oils are, it is a massive 265 pounds of peppermint leaves for just one pound of the essential oil. That's a powerfully concentrated oil! Due to the level of concentration, you will only require only a tiny amount of oil. Additionally, nearly all essential oils need to be dilute to avoid contact with skin.

Certain essential oils like lemon, orange grapefruit, lime, grapefruit, and bergamot - can cause skin to become less sensitive to sun (UV sunlight). This is referred to as photosensitivity. It can lead to skin discoloration and blisters. skin. It also makes your skin more prone to sunburn. To avoid photosensitivity, do not apply any essential oils that can cause this issue within 12 hours in which your skin is exposed to the sun's rays.

The majority of experts recommend that you do not use essential oils on infants or children unless you have approval from a respected doctor. If you decide to use essential oils for your little ones, be sure to use extreme care in diluting the oil in a greater way than you would do for an adult. The skin of infants and children is more sensitive than adults, and oil that is safe may harm the skin of children and babies. But, there are few essential oils that doctors have agreed are safe, if utilized correctly, on children and babies. They include chamomile lavender, frankincense and orange. However you shouldn't make use of eucalyptus or peppermint rosemary, or wintergreen essential oils on children and babies.

www.ingramcontent.com/pod-product-compliance
Lightning Source LLC
Chambersburg PA
CBHW060333030426
42336CB00011B/1321